Pray for Valerie! (KNEE)
MY FITNESS PAL (APP)

W9-AAT-577

In *Bod4God*, Steve Reynolds launches a full-scale frontal assault in the ongoing American war with obesity. His weapons—solid biblical teaching and modern fitness principles—serve more effectively than any smart bomb or stealth warplane in this battle. Reynolds's easy-to-understand, motivating plan can help even the most sedentary couch potato and is especially effective because it uses eternal wisdom from God's Word. Read *Bod4God* today and enlist in the healthy army of the fit and faithful!

DARREN BARONI, MD
Member of American College of Gastroenterology
Attending Gastroenterologist

Americans are in a fight for their health against a formidable "Goliath": obesity. For years, the scientific community has told us what "stones" will weaken the giant: good nutrition and exercise. But translating bench-top research to everyday living is the challenge. In *Bod4God*, Pastor Reynolds teaches us to be the "David." Armed with the slingshot of God's Word, you will launch healthy, up-to-date, scientific principles of exercise and nutrition to fight head-on the epidemic of obesity and topple the giant!

ELIZABETH P. BERBANO, MD, MPH
Fellow of the American College of Physicians
Certified, American Board of Internal Medicine

It's been a blessing to partner with Pastor Reynolds and his congregation to provide Body & Soul as a key exercise strategy for the Bod4God program. In *Bod4God* there is a place for everyone to be successful. People of all ages and fitness levels have participated and seen improvements in cardiovascular fitness, strength and flexibility. You will be encouraged and empowered by this book as you seek to improve your health and live a life of energy and vitality to God's glory.

JEANNIE BLOCHER
President, Body & Soul Fitness Ministries
Certified Faculty, American Council on Exercise
Group Fitness Specialist, Ken Cooper's Institute, Dallas, Texas

One area of teaching that seems to be neglected in the Church today is the area of our own health. The Bible tells us our bodies are the temple of the Holy Spirit, but do we really treat our bodies with that value in mind? That's why I'm so excited about *Bod4God*. Steve brings biblical principles to bear to help everyone with weight loss, exercise and staying healthy. Every Christian should read this book—now!

JONATHAN FALWELL
Pastor, Thomas Road Baptist Church, Lynchburg, Virginia

Bod4God has produced more sustainable weight loss for its participants than any other program that I have been involved with in my 20 years as a dietitian. The focus on God and on losing weight for the right reasons was genuinely inspiring. The bonding, trust and support of other participants helped keep the momentum going to achieve truly impressive results. Pastor Steve Reynolds is a great living example of God's power to transform.

VIVIAN HUTSON, MA, MHA, RD, LD, FACHE
Registered Dietician

I have seen patients turn life-threatening conditions into manageable ones or even experience full restoration through lifestyle change, including diet and exercise. Pastor Reynolds shows the powerful effects of faith and lifestyle change in his transformation from an obese man to a man unburdened by weight and illness.

ULRICH PRINZ, MD
Board-certified Internist

Bod4God is a much-needed reminder that God created our bodies as tools for His work and, as such, His Word has plenty to say about how we treat them. I first met Steve when he joined my coaching network, and I have been impressed with his insights. We would all be wise to take his words to heart. After all, our bodies are the handiwork of God, meant to aid us in carrying His message to the world. Without health, none of us can be very effective. Kudos to Steve for bringing this issue out of the dark!

NELSON SEARCY
Lead Pastor of The Journey Church in New York City
Founder of www.ChurchLeaderInsights.com

Pastor Reynolds is a modern day prophet who strikes at the heart of the unhealthy lifestyle of most Americans and many members of the Christian community. His biblically based *Bod4God* is a credible program that could spark a movement toward weight control and healthier living. I heartily endorse this well-written, exciting book.

JAMES M. STERN, MD
Fellow of the American College of Surgeons

Steve Reynolds has a great spirit of discipline and commitment to Jesus Christ, which is reflected in this book. For those who want to lose weight, you should read *Bod4God* to catch the *spirit*—just not the practical lessons, but the spiritual lessons as well. Steve has put the right priority in weight loss—a person's relationship to God—and from that discipline concerning the "temple of the Holy Spirit" they can lose weight.

ELMER L. TOWNS
Cofounder, Liberty University
Author of the bestselling *Fasting for Spiritual Breakthrough*

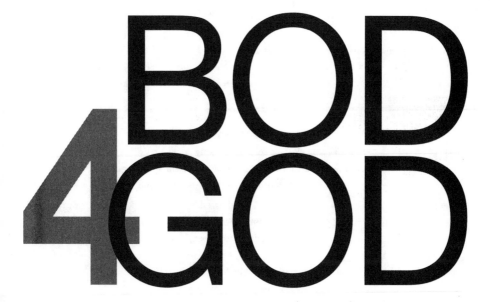

BOD 4 GOD

The Four Keys to Weight Loss

STEVE REYNOLDS

Regal

From Gospel Light
Ventura, California, U.S.A.

Published by Regal
From Gospel Light
Ventura, California, U.S.A.
www.regalbooks.com
Printed in the U.S.A.

Library of Congress Cataloging-in-Publication Data
Reynolds, Steve, Pastor.
Bod4God : the four keys to weight loss / Steve Reynolds.
p. cm.
ISBN 978-0-8307-5157-0 (hard cover)
1. Weight loss. 2. Weight loss—Religious aspects—Christianity.
3. Health—Religious aspects—Christianity. 4. Reducing diets. I. Title.
RM222.2.R465 2009
613.2'5—dc22
2009033951

Rights for publishing this book outside the U.S.A. or in non-English languages are
administered by Gospel Light Worldwide, an international not-for-profit ministry.
For additional information, please visit www.glww.org, email info@glww.org, or write to
Gospel Light Worldwide, 1957 Eastman Avenue, Ventura, CA 93003, U.S.A.

*First, I dedicate this book to my God, who is the source
of my life. I will spend the rest of my days on this earth
honoring You with my body.*

*"According to my earnest expectation and hope that in nothing
I shall be ashamed, but with all boldness, as always, so now also Christ
will be magnified in my body, whether by life or by death."*
PHILIPPIANS 1:20

*Second, I dedicate this book to Debbie, my wife, who is
my partner in life. I will spend the rest of my days on this earth
loving you with my body.*

*"Who can find a virtuous wife? For her worth is far above rubies.
The heart of her husband safely trusts her; so he will have no lack of gain.
She does him good and not evil all the days of her life. Her husband is
known in the gates, when he sits among the elders of the land."*
PROVERBS 31:10-12,23

*Third, I dedicate this book to Crystal, Sarah and Jeremiah,
my children, who are the inspiration for my life. I will spend the
rest of my days influencing you with my body.*

"I have no greater joy than to hear that my children walk in truth."
3 JOHN 1:4

Contents

Acknowledgments

This was a TEAM project.

I greatly appreciate the group of people who helped me develop this book, including:

My parents, for always supporting me. I love you both very much.

My family, for sacrificing time without your husband and father while I worked on this book.

My church family, members and staff of Capital Baptist Church in Annandale, Virginia, for your loyal support. It is truly an honor to serve as your pastor.

My colaborers, the leaders and participants in the Losing to Live Weight Loss Competitions throughout the country and the world. Your partnership is invaluable in the ongoing success of this movement.

My pastor, the late Jerry Falwell, for your impact on my life and ministry. I miss you!

My mentor Elmer Towns, cofounder of Liberty University, and my friend Carole Lewis, Director of First Place 4 Health, for assistance in advancing this book.

My friends Gary and Jana Moritz, for your creative contribution to this project.

My writing assistant, Gwen Ellis—thank you for all you did to help this busy pastor.

My photographer, Randy Ritter, who took most of the pictures in this book.

My publisher, Regal Books, and especially Kim Bangs, for your guidance in producing a quality book.

My media contacts—thank you for helping to spread the Bod4God message around the country and the world.

My readers—you honor me for taking time out of your busy lives to read this book.

Foreword

By Carole Lewis

I met Steve Reynolds in 2007, when he invited me to speak at one of his Losing to Live Orientations. I was thrilled to walk into the sanctuary of Steve's church and to see that there were so many men who were interested in losing weight and pursuing a healthier lifestyle. Steve has been hosting the Losing to Live competition at his church for the last two years, and the participants have lost more than 6,000 pounds.

There are many things I admire about Steve Reynolds, but number one on the list is that he is a pastor who has lost 100 pounds after struggling with his weight for many years. Steve told me that his church members would have surely confronted him if he got drunk every week, but his weighing more than 300 pounds was never challenged because being overweight is acceptable in the Christian community today.

After being diagnosed with Type II diabetes, Steve became concerned that he might not live long enough to see his daughters married with children of their own. Steve knew that God was interested in this part of his life and that God was only too willing to help him if he would just begin eating less and exercising. Steve began to study what the Bible has to say about taking care of our bodies and found that it has a lot to say on the subject.

Another thing that I admire about Steve Reynolds is his love and concern for other pastors and their congregations who are in poor health and unable to serve God effectively because of their excess weight and sedentary lifestyles. Steve believes, as I do, that focusing solely on weight loss usually leads to failure. The only way for a person to truly succeed is to change his or her lifestyle. Through the Losing to Live competitions that Steve conducts in his own church, he helps individuals make simple changes in their eating and exercising habits to get on the right track, while being encouraged by others in the program. Steve believes that fitness is not a fad—it's a forever life plan—and details the plan in this book.

Steve's concern is for the health of Christians, the health of our churches and the health of our nation. Obesity is one of the major health problems in our country today. Kids are obese. Their parents are obese. Their grandparents are obese. We are all killing ourselves with a knife and fork. Coronary heart disease, Type II diabetes, cancers, hypertension, stroke, liver disease, gallbladder disease, sleep apnea, respiratory problems, osteoarthritis and gynecological problems including infertility can all be directly related to obesity. Over the last few years, legislators have tried to find some way to curb this morbid obesity, but it takes more than legislation to fix the problem: It also takes personal commitment.

When you consider the risks of obesity, why wouldn't you run—not walk—to a place where you could sit down, read this book, make weight-loss a top priority and begin to change so that you could live? What you eat and whether you exercise are personal choices, but these are personal choices that affect all of us in terms of health care costs and quality of life. Steve believes it is a tough go for people to lose weight on their own, but with God's help and the encouragement of a group of like-minded weight losers, anyone can become healthier and live a full rich life.

Before You Begin

A Word from Pastor Steve

You've picked up this book because you have a need to lose weight—or at least you have an interest in losing weight. Maybe you're tired of endless weight-loss plans and endless years of trying to get the numbers on that scale to start moving downward. Maybe you are feeling as if this is your last attempt to find something that will work. You've come to the right place. I can help you.

I understand what you've been through, because I've been through it too. I understand how frustrated you've become, because I've been frustrated too. Perhaps, like me, you've heard frightening news from your doctor who has warned you to lose weight—now!

First of all, I want you to know that not only do I understand your situation, but I also care about it. I care about you. I've become so passionate about turning overweight people into losers that much of my life today is wrapped up in finding ways to help people change. I was a fat little kid who grew up, played football through college, vowed never to exercise again after I quit playing football, kept the promise and ballooned to a weight of 340 pounds. I heard my own doctor say those fearful words, "You have diabetes." Even then, it took me a while to begin doing something about my obesity.

Then, with God's help, I found a way to begin taking small steps, and those small steps led to a new lifestyle. They led to life. That's what this book is all about—a path to a new life. I want to share what I've learned, because it works. I've lost more than 100 pounds and am still losing. I no longer need medications for my diabetes. I now control it through my diet. Now I really feel good and have lots of energy. I'll share my secrets with you—all of them. You won't find them very profound or complicated, but I can promise you that if you start taking what I call "Small Steps to Life," and you stick with them, they will work for you as they have for others who've been through our weight-loss challenge at our church, Capital Baptist Church.

What Is "Losing to Live"?

Christians are the most overweight people group in America. Losing to Live has been designed to confront and solve this problem. There are two ways to approach weight-loss using this program: as a personal challenge or as a group competition. Losing to Live will show you how to lose weight and keep it off through establishing a Bod4God lifestyle. There are four keys to weight loss. They are:

1. **D**edication: Honoring God with Your Body
2. **I**nspiration: Motivating Yourself for Change
3. **E**at and Exercise: Managing Your Habits
4. **T**eam: Building Your Circle of Support

See, I told you these four keys are not very complex! But they work, and they have made a better body possible for thousands of people. They can do the same thing for you.

Three Reasons "Losing to Live" Will Work for You

There are three unique aspects of Losing to Live that make it so effective. They are:

1. It is *biblical*. You will learn how to apply the Bible to your life in the area of losing weight and improving your health.
2. It is *personal*. You will learn how to craft your own individual lifestyle plan.
3. It is *incremental*. You will learn how to choose "Small Steps to Life" that will slowly but surely lead you to lasting life change.

This powerful combination is what will make this plan so successful for you.

What It Takes to Be a Big Loser

The Bod4God Victory Guide at the end of each chapter is the place where you will take the information in this book and make it personal in your life. It includes the weekly memory verse, reflection/application questions and the "Small Steps to Life" record. The thorough completion of these things will equip you to practice the four keys to weight loss. Big losers make the Victory Guide a high priority!

So, are you ready for a weight-loss program that really works? Will you take the 12 weeks to a better body challenge? Then join the Losing to Live weight-loss program, and before you know it, you will have a Bod4God.

Blessings on you,
Pastor Steve Reynolds

Pastor Steve Before

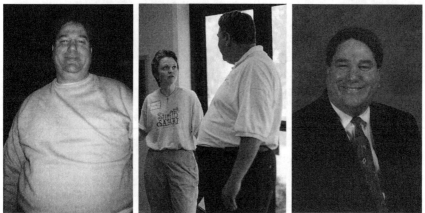

Pastor Steve After

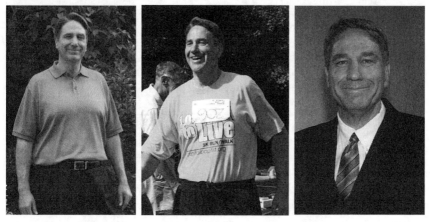

BOD 4 GOD

Celebrate and monitor your accomplishments as you complete the weekly Victory Guide assignments at the end of each chapter by putting a checkmark in the designated box.

VICTORY GUIDE CHART

Week	Read *Bod4God* Chapter	Memory Verse	Answer Questions	Do Small Steps to Life	Record My Progress Report
1	The Anti-Fat Pastor	Col. 1:16			
2	Losing to Live	Matt. 16:24-25			
3	*D* Is for Dedication	Gal. 5:16			
4	*D* Is for More Dedication	Rom. 10:9			
5	*I* Is for Inspiration	John 10:10			
6	*I* Is for More Inspiration	Phil. 4:13			
7	*E* Is for Eat	1 Thess. 4:4			
8	*E* Is for Exercise	1 Cor. 10:31			
9	*T* Is for Team: A Personal Challenge	Ps. 51:12			
10	*T* Is for Team: A Group Competition	Eccles. 4:9			
11	Frequently Asked Questions	1 Pet. 3:15			
12	Your Lifestyle Plan	Review			

The Anti-fat Pastor

For by him all things were created that are in heaven and that are on earth,
visible and invisible, whether thrones or dominions or principalities or powers.
All things were created through Him and for Him.

Colossians 1:16

Calling the Flock to God, Away from the Fridge:
Northern Virginia Pastor Joins Ranks of Faithful Eyeing Scales
The Washington Post, Monday, January 22, 2007

There it was in bold print and on the front page of the Washington Post, and it was about me—me, Steve Reynolds, a local pastor who got sick and tired of being sick and tired and decided to do something about it, starting with losing weight. It's a long story. So let's rewind to the beginning, back to where weight began to be a problem for me.

I grew up in a Southern blue-collar family in a small town. My background was very simple. My parents didn't graduate from high school. No one in our family had ever graduated from college until my brother and I did. But here I was, pastor of a church in suburban Washington, D. C., and dealing with my own weight problem, when all of a sudden I wind up on the front page of a major metropolitan newspaper, the *Washington Post*. I'm definitely not a front-page-of-the-paper kind of guy. First came the article and then came many interviews, including one with Neil Cavuto of Fox News. Neil is the first person to label me as the "Anti-Fat" pastor.

I had struggled with weight all of my life. In first grade, when most kids weigh about 45 pounds, I weighed more than a hundred—104 to be exact. My mother said that when I was a baby, I had a super-sensitive stomach. I had a tough time keeping food down, but Mom must have succeeded in getting some of the food to stay down because I began to pack on weight.

I'm proud of my Southern heritage, but you probably know about the traditional Southern diet. I ate a lot of fried chicken, pecan pie, sweet tea—lots of grease and sugar in my food. My diet was as unhealthy as it could be. It's not uncommon to see overweight kids today, but in 1963, it was rather unusual, and I looked unusual. I really stood out in the class picture. Mom had to shop in the "husky boys" clothing section of the store. I wasn't just a little bit overweight; I had childhood obesity. By the time I started being concerned about my weight, I'd been overweight for many years.

Throughout much of my life, I thought I was just fine. I even poked fun at people who were lean and fit. I'd say things like, "Where's the beef, skinny guy? Real men eat red meat," and "Who, me? Eat salad? Salads are for sissies." Probably, if the truth were told, I was covering up for a low self-image. Most overweight people do.

In grade school, I started playing sports. I was a big kid; and at that time, kids were ranked first by age and then by weight. The coaches would ask, "How old are you?" "Eight," I'd answer. Then, because my weight was far above the weight set for kids my age, and because I might hurt some of the smaller eight-year-olds when playing with them, I was bumped up to the next division. I had to play with older kids. There were times when I was bumped up two divisions. I never did play with kids my own age.

In some ways, being in a higher division worked to my advantage from the standpoint that I became a pretty good football player and got offers from half-a-dozen small colleges. I accepted one at Liberty University in Virginia. I was a four-year starter on Liberty's football team, and I was fortunate to go through college on a full football scholarship. I thank the Lord for that scholarship, but to keep and develop my football skills and my strength, I had to stay active throughout the year. College football was, and is, a year-round sport. That helped me maintain a good weight.

I started playing football when I was about eight years old, and I played all the way through until I was 22. Then, when I finished, I made myself a promise. "Nobody's ever going to make me exercise again for the rest of my life." I was sick of everything associated with playing football—the push-ups, the running, the exhaustion, the pain, the pressure. I've broken plenty of promises in my life, but unfortunately, I kept this one. I quit exercising. You know what happened. I started putting on weight.

When I graduated from college, I went on to seminary. I ate what I wanted to eat, and I kept my promise not to exercise. After seminary, I was ordained, and my beautiful bride, Debbie, and I were excited about our future together. We felt called to be church planters. In the fall of 1982, I launched a new church plant just outside Washington, DC. I soon learned that only 1 of 10 new churches becomes successfully established; 90 percent fail. *Hmm.* I had just begun to work in a field with a 90-percent failure rate. I don't like to fail, and I wasn't about to fail at establishing this church. I was determined to work as hard as I could to make this church plant successful. I wanted my tombstone to read, "Here is a man who prayed like it all depended on God, and worked like it all depended on him."

The good news is the church started to grow; the bad news is, so did I. I worked as hard as I could during the day. I knocked on doors and contacted people about our new church. No one had asked me to come here and start a church, so I had to go out and let people know about it. When I came home late in the evening, I'd sit down in my La-Z-Boy recliner. (I've worn out three chairs so far in my life and I plan to go to the grave still owning some kind of La-Z-Boy chair.) A real man has a La-Z-Boy chair, and when I'm in mine, I hold the remote. Anybody can sit in my chair and hold the remote when I'm not home, but when I come in, you need to get out of my chair and hand over the remote so nobody will get hurt. So as soon as I'd greeted my family, I'd get into my chair and start eating.

I've even thought about bringing my chair to church and doing a series on things I've learned sitting in my chair. One of the things I learned and could teach for sure is how to eat ice cream. Late at night, in that La-Z-Boy, I ate every kind of food in general, and ice cream in particular. I loved ice cream. I was truly *addicted* to it. I ate it every night. I had seen the ice cream eating pattern modeled every day of my childhood, and we are shaped by what we see modeled for us. To this day, my dad eats ice cream every night. I've seen him polish off a half-gallon of ice cream at a time. Dad, however, is only a little overweight because he walks regularly. I, on the other hand, faithfully kept my promise never to exercise again.

I had worked at a grocery store for years, so when Debbie and I got married, I volunteered to do the grocery shopping for our family. I still shop for the family's groceries. When I went shopping for food, I'd search for ice cream that was on sale and then buy six half-gallons at a time. As church planters, we were struggling financially, but I had to have my ice cream. I'd go down the aisle looking for whatever was on sale. When Breyer's chocolate chip was on sale, that was especially exciting. I didn't know if the kids were going to have Pampers, but no matter how tough times were, I was going to have my ice cream. Here I was, not exercising and eating whatever I wanted. I grew and grew and grew to 340 pounds. I had terrible health: high blood pressure, high cholesterol and diabetes. I was literally digging my grave with a knife, fork, and, of course, an ice cream spoon.

Diabetes will kill you. The disease runs in my family, and while I hoped I'd never get it, I wasn't too surprised when I was diagnosed with it. I didn't ask what I could do to change the situation. I didn't even consider a lifestyle change. I just looked at the doctor and asked, "What pills do I need to take to control this?" He gave me prescriptions and I began taking eight pills a day for the diabetes and other health-related problems.

This went on for six years. Then I heard that if you lose weight it might help to control diabetes. I learned that losing weight could also help control high blood pressure, high cholesterol and a number of other illnesses, some of which I already had. Diabetes is not always a weight-related issue, and I wouldn't want anyone reading this book to start trying to lose weight and stop taking insulin. If you have diabetes, you need to work carefully with your medical doctor to monitor your condition.

Diabetes can also be hereditary. My grandfather was a skinny, muscular farmer who was probably never overweight a day in his life, *and* he was a diabetic. My mother is a diabetic who *is* overweight. Well, I had diabetes *and* I was definitely overweight. *Would I be able to control my diabetes if I lost weight?* I wondered.

God had begun to work in my heart, and He was telling me I needed to do something about my overeating and lack of exercise. Slowly, I began the journey of trying to improve my health. At first, the issue was so personal that I told no one. I kept it between God and me. I knew I could never lose weight and be fit without God's intervention. I began to pray and seek His direction. I started losing weight, and when I had lost 70 pounds, my diabetes and other problems were brought under control. To this day, I'm free from those illnesses.

God is faithful, and He is able. He led me to a passage in His Word that directly addresses the issues I was facing. It was the Colossians passage at the beginning of this chapter. I learned that everything that exists was created by Him and for Him. That included me. If He was in control of all things, then He was in control of my life, and if I'd let Him, He could be in control of my weight issues too. It was a wonderful revelation!

As I prayed and meditated on this Scripture, God gave me a step-by-step prescription for making a huge change in my life—a change I'm going to share in the pages of this book. Once I began to follow it, I began to see results. Yes, I saw physical changes, but I also saw spiritual changes. My faith increased with each change I made and each pound I shed. I knew I'd discovered something important and it was my responsibility to share what I'd learned with my church and my community. I realized that Christians are the most overweight people group on earth.[1] We are more overweight than Muslims, Hindus, Buddhists and every other religion you can name. (More about this later.)

Christians should be the most healthy people group, especially when we consider the physical condition of Jesus Christ, our Founder and Leader. Carole Lewis is an author and the director of a successful weight-loss program called "First Place 4 Health," so-called because as Christians, we are to give Christ first place in our lives and that means in all things, even what we put in our mouths. She said, "The pictures of Jesus that I remember from my childhood showed Him to be rather frail; however, the Jesus of the Scriptures is quite a different person. We know that Jesus was a carpenter by trade. Until He began His public ministry at age 30, He earned His living as a carpenter. He had to carry large pieces of wood and stone to build structures. His trade required great physical strength. We also know from Scripture that Jesus walked from Sidon to Tyre, which would have been a 40-mile trip [that He could have walked] in one day."[2]

Little Christs

When God spoke to me about my weight, I finally faced my situation. I took the first step. I decided to go to the Bible for help. Philippians 1:20-21 says, "Christ will be magnified in my body, whether by life or by death. For to me, to live is Christ, and to die is gain." Christ wanted to be magnified in my body! That was amazing!

I'm a Christian, and "Christian" means "little Christ." In other words, we are to be Christ-like. Our Leader—Jesus Christ—was in such great physical condition that He could walk 40 miles, not in Reeboks but in leather sandals; and yet His followers on this planet are unhealthy, overweight, sedentary couch potatoes. That concerns me, and it ought to concern you. God wants to address this condition not only in our bodies but in our churches as well. God wants to help us in this area of weight management.

What the Bible Says

Colossians 1:16 says that "all things were created through Him and for Him." That means everything in heaven, everything on earth, everything visible and everything invisible. He set up thrones, dominions, rulers and authorities. Everything that exists has been created *by* Christ and *for* Him . . . even your body. God is your Creator. He has given you life. We Christians are strong on the Creator aspect of God's character, but we are weak in the area of a God who is also our Controller. He must also be the Controller of our life. If we are made for God, then our body belongs to God. And that's what this program is all about.

The word "body" is found 179 times in the Bible. I started studying those passages. Approximately one-third of them talk about our future body in heaven. It will be perfect and will not be affected by what we eat or don't eat—including ice cream. We will have a heavenly body; but today, we are still living in an earthly body. I started studying the remaining Scripture references to body. Out of my study, God showed me the four keys to a better body. As I mentioned, those keys are:

- **D**edication: Honoring God with Your Body
- **I**nspiration: Motivating Yourself for Change
- **E**at and Exercise: Managing Your Habits
- **T**eam: Building Your Circle of Support

Then God helped me apply those keys and I started losing weight. People noticed and began to ask what plan I was on to lose weight. I had so many people ask me what I was doing that I decided to do a sermon series on getting a body for God. I called it "Bod4God."

I'm a Loser

Four times a year I send out a card listing my sermon series. One of those times in 2007, I put the Bod4God topic on the card. Thousands of people got the mailing, including a reporter from the *Washington Post*. She called me and said, "Pastor, I got the postcard and it sounds pretty interesting. A church talking about weight loss? That's a little unusual. I'd like to come hear those messages." Of course I invited her to come. She came and wrote the article we talked about earlier. I expected it to appear on some back page of the *Washington Post*. However, there it was, right on the front page. The article was picked up by the Associated Press and literally went all over the world. I knew then that God was up to something. Then came the Fox News interview and a lot of others, and I became the "Anti-Fat Pastor."

Today, I am proud to announce that I'm a loser. I'm proud that I've lost more than 100 pounds. My diabetes is controlled by lifestyle. While I understand that not every diabetic can control the disease by losing weight, it has worked for me and I am thankful. I know that someday the diabetes might return since it is in my family genetics; but for now, I don't have it.

I would like nothing better than to see whole churches full of losers. My goal at my church—Capital Baptist Church—is to be the greatest losing church in America. What about you? What about your church? I'm not here to judge anyone or any church about weight. I still need to lose more weight myself, and since I have struggled with weight all my life, I know the difficult part for me will be keeping the weight off. I'll struggle with it to the end of my days, but I am confident that by applying all that I present to you in this book, I can keep the weight off.

"Small Steps to Life" Will Work for You

Losing weight may seem impossible to you. Perhaps you've tried every diet plan known to man and none have worked. One of the main reasons those fad diets don't work is that they ask you to do too much too soon. When that happens, you get frustrated and quit. I understand; so I want to encourage you to start with "Small Steps to Life" that you can do. If you just do a few steps in the areas of eating and exercising the first week, and then you are faithful to do those steps every day, the following week you will be able to add more steps that will help you gradually move toward weight-loss success. What you are building is a new lifestyle—one that will be filled with health and energy.

In this program, the difference between weight loss and no weight loss is based on what you do about creating "Small Steps to Life." People who consistently implement these small steps will lose weight; those who don't implement any small steps will not lose weight.

Pastor Steve's "Small Steps to Life"

To get started on my weight-loss and healthy body quest, I consistently took this small spiritual step to life:

I had (and continue to have) a special time with God every day to fill up the inner man. He truly is my portion (see Ps. 119:57). When my inner man has been stuffed full, my physical man won't be so hungry, and I will have better control over what I eat.

Here are some of the food substitution small steps that worked for me:

- Instead of a bagel, I eat a protein health bar
- Instead of ice cream, I eat nonfat yogurt
- Instead of diet sodas, I drink water during the day
- I went from eating no fruit to eating an apple a day
- I went from eating a hamburger and fries to eating chicken salad with a small amount of lowfat dressing
- Instead of using mayonnaise on sandwiches, I use mustard
- Instead of fried chips and dip, I eat baked chips and salsa
- Instead of eating lots of beef, I eat lots of chicken and some fish
- Instead of white bread, I eat whole-grain bread
- Instead of fried foods, I eat baked foods (reduces the amount of fat)
- Instead of vegetable oil, I use olive oil (a monounsaturated oil—the good kind of fat!)
- Instead of high-fat creamer, I use fat-free creamer
- I went from taking no vitamins to taking daily vitamins
- I went from eating no kale to eating lots of kale (a dark green, highly nutritious vegetable)
- I went from eating no blueberries to eating lots of blueberries (a powerful antioxidant food)
- I stopped eating canned food (can contain lots of salt and preservatives) to eating fresh or frozen food
- I went from eating peanut butter and crackers to eating almonds (a good source of protein and monounsaturated fat)
- I went from using Sweet 'n' Low to using Stevia (a sweetener that has a negligible effect on blood glucose levels)
- I stopped eating mostly processed foods to eating whole, unprocessed foods
- I went from taking in no flaxseed to eating ground flaxseed on cereals, salads, in drinks, and so on (good for heart health and cholesterol levels)

To get started with exercise, I intentionally moved more. I would go out of my way to walk farther and put more effort in my daily activities.

I then went to the gym and started walking on the treadmill and lifting weights. I started slowly, and gradually increased my time on the treadmill and my weight-training repetitions.

Your "Small Steps to Life"

Now it's your turn to craft your own individual lifestyle plan. Throughout this book, you will find some ideas for "Small Steps to Life." These ideas may or may not work for you. You must research activities and ways to move that you will enjoy, and discover healthy habits that you can do for the rest of your life. Start slowly and increase activity gradually; but above all, be consistent. Over a period of time, your small steps will take you a great distance.

Notes

1. Ken Ferraro, "Study Finds Some Faithful Less Likely to Pass the Plate. ferraro@purdue.edu, http://news.uns.purdue.edu.
2. Carole Lewis, *Choosing to Change* (Ventura, CA: Regal Books, 2001), p. 20.
3. These are general guidelines for water consumption. However, there are certain circumstances when an individual may be on medications or have underlying kidney disease or other chronic illness in which "too much" water is detrimental to health. As with any general health guidelines, please consult with your personal physician or health care provider for specific recommendations based upon your medication profile, health history and level of exercise.

Small Steps to Life Ideas

What Do You Need to Know About H_2O?

You must drink an adequate amount of water to be healthy and lose weight; so every week I am going to give you a little more information about water's importance. Every weight-loss program advocates drinking more water than most of us drink on a regular basis. Why? Many times we are not hungry, but thirsty. Our brain interprets thirst as hunger, and we start grazing for something to satisfy the body's need. The Mayo Clinic website on the subject of how much water to drink says that we need to replace the fluids our body loses each day. The average output of urine is about 6.3 cups per day for an adult. In addition, other bodily processes such as breathing and sweating account for additional fluid loss. Fluid loss must be replaced on a daily basis. Eight 8-ounce glasses of water a day will cover your body's need for fluid unless you are perspiring heavily due to exercise or hot weather.

There are some schools of thought that say you need to take your weight and divide it in half. That's the amount of water (in ounces) that you should be drinking each day. Perhaps you are among those who say they don't like to drink water. That's because you have never tried it. Once you start drinking enough water, your body will crave it and will respond positively to being well hydrated.

There is a debate about whether other fluids such as soft drinks, fruit juice and iced teas should be counted as water intake. While they are liquid, anything with caffeine in it acts as a diuretic and further strips water from your system. Fruit juices and tea with sugar—natural or added sugar—are processed by the body as food. The best solution is to drink plain water and drink enough so that you rarely feel thirsty and your urine is only slightly yellow.

Do this one small step of drinking more water each day, and stay with it. It *will* make a difference. Since our intent is to build a new lifestyle, drinking enough water is a good way to begin.[3]

Small Food Step

I began to get control of my eating by portion-controlled eating. Remember, your stomach is about the size of your fist, so don't eat the size of your head. Your approach should be to slowly and systematically decrease the unhealthy things you are eating and slowly and systematically increase the good things you should be eating. This approach works because it allows you to retrain your taste buds and develop the right food cravings.

Small Exercise Step

Walk more. Park your car at the far perimeter of the shopping center and walk to the stores in that complex rather than parking close and moving your car every time you change stores. Although this is an incredibly small thing, it will get you started on a larger exercise program.

Small Steps to Life Record

What "Skinny Things" Will You Do this Week?

Fill out this chart each week by indicating: (1) What you will do to eat less to live; (2) What you will do to exercise more to live; and (3) What average daily ounces of water you will drink. Pick only a few things, and stick with them. Remember that weight loss and maintenance requires you to *eat less* and *exercise more*.

Sun.	
Mon.	
Tues.	
Wed.	
Thurs.	
Fri.	
Sat.	

Bod4God Victory Guide

The Bod4God Victory Guide at the end of each chapter is where you will take the information in this book and make it personal in your life. It includes the weekly memory verse, reflection/application questions, small steps to life record and journal. Your thorough completion of these things will equip you to practice the four keys to weight loss. Big losers make the Victory Guide a high priority. Each week, record your weight change on "My Progress Report" located in appendix A.

Week One: The Anti-Fat Pastor

Memory Verse
"For by Him all things were created that are in heaven and that are on earth, visible and invisible, whether thrones or dominions or principalities or powers. All things were created through Him and for Him" (Col. 1:16).

Reflection/Application Questions
1. Notice the two ways you were created in Colossians 1:16: through God and for God. What does it mean to you to be created by God? What does it mean to you to be created for God?

   _____

   _____

   _____

   _____

   _____

2. In what ways do you think this verse is related to your struggle to get your weight under control and become healthier?

   _____

   _____

   _____

   _____

   _____

3. How much of a role, if any, has your childhood and social culture played in your struggle with weight?

_____

_____

_____

_____

4. In this chapter, I make a connection between the bad habits I learned from my family growing up and the behaviors I developed on my own. Note that I am careful not to place the blame on my family for the struggles I have had with my weight as an adult. Which of the following might you be tempted to blame for your struggle with weight?

____ Parents   ____ Metabolism   ____ Genetics

____ Stress   ____ Heritage   ____ Gender

____ God   ____ Self   ____ Stage of Life

____ Occupation   ____ Environment   ____ Finances

____ Other: _____

5. Two of the habits that put me in the situation of being severely overweight included my nightly routines of La-Z-Boy lounging and eating ice cream. What are some habits that have negatively impacted your health?

_____

_____

_____

_____

6. Developing diabetes and my deep desire to live was my motivation to lose weight and lead a healthier lifestyle. What is your motivation for physical change?

_____

_____

_____

_____

7. How would you assess your past attempts to lose weight and get healthy? What did you do to make your weight go up or down?

_____

_____

_____

_____

_____

_____

8. Think about the times when you lost or gained a major amount of weight. What was going on in your life at that time? School activities? Marriage? A new baby? A career or job change? The death of a friend, a family member or a pet? Write down what you did in response to these events that caused your weight to go up or down.

_____

_____

_____

_____

_____

_____

My Bod4God Journal

Teach me, O Lord, the way of Your statutes, and I shall keep it to the end.
PSALM 119:33

Record what God is telling you to do this week to apply the four keys to a better body.

Dedication: Honoring God with My Body

_____
_____
_____
_____
_____

Inspiration: Motivating Myself for Change

_____
_____
_____
_____
_____

Eat and Exercise: Managing My Habits

_____
_____
_____
_____

Team: Building My Circle of Support

_____
_____
_____
_____
_____

Losing to Live

Then Jesus said to His disciples, "If anyone desires to come after Me, let him deny himself, and take up his cross, and follow Me. For whoever desires to save his life will lose it, but whoever loses his life for My sake will find it."

MATTHEW 16:24-25

This passage of Scripture is repeated six times in the Bible. Jesus made this statement to multiple people in multiple places. It was a major theme of His preaching. Everywhere He went, He wanted people to know, "Hey, you want life? Who doesn't? Here's how you get it. Deny yourself, take up your cross, and follow me." God burned this passage into my heart. It has probably had more influence on my life than any other passage of Scripture. For me, incorporating this passage into my life became the challenge of losing weight so that I could live—I call it "losing to live."

God created our bodies, and He created them for himself. Your body is the temple of the Holy Spirit. It is a holy place. You may ask, "Is God really concerned about my body?" Well, He's concerned enough that He mentions the word "body" 179 times in the Bible. When He deals with something that many times, it's important! The good news is that because our body is so important, God gives us instructions regarding how to take care of it. He tells us how we can honor Him with our body. Since God considers our body important, we should too.

God made us in His image. Wow! Think of it. It is truly awesome to have the image of the living God within us. God gave us everything we would ever need to live on this earth. Man is His crowning achievement. When man sinned and fell from grace, God gave us the best that heaven had to offer so that we could be redeemed. He gave us His only Son,

Jesus. He also sent His Holy Spirit, not only to comfort us, but also to indwell us. God has a huge vested interest in us, His creation. Doesn't it follow, then, that we need to take care of the body He has given us? Doesn't it make sense that our bodies should be finely tuned instruments fit for His use? We will honor Him by having a Bod4God lifestyle.

More Than a Weight-Loss Plan

In this book, I'm telling you how I lost more than 100 pounds. However, the book isn't just about losing weight. It's about taking small steps to change your lifestyle that will put you on a path to health for the rest of your life. I call these "Small Steps to Life." You'll move from eating food that is killing you to eating food that will build your body's strength. You'll move from being a couch potato to being physically active. You'll move from being unhealthy to being physically fit.

A very important question to ask yourself is this: "Is the way I'm living and feeling now the way I want to live and feel five years from now? Ten years from now? Twenty years from now? Is this the way I want to spend the rest of my life?" Think about how you might look and feel in a few years if you don't make changes now. Is that what you really want for your life? Do you honestly think that without making changes you will suddenly become healthy, be able to play with your kids and grandkids, put in a full day of physical activity and be alert and engaged with others? Or do you see yourself plopped down more or less permanently in that La-Z-Boy recliner? Maybe without making changes you won't have the health issues that I had, but there are many other illnesses that are the direct result of obesity (more about that in Chapter 9).

God says that as our days are, so shall our strength be (see Deut. 33:25). As long as we are on this planet, God has work for us to do. He has much that needs to be done for His kingdom, and He is looking for those who are willing and equipped to do that work. "Equipped" means having a body that can do what He needs it to do. At age 50, Albert Schweitzer was finally able to begin His missionary medical practice in Africa after retraining in medicine at age 40, and after being interned as a prisoner of war. Mother Teresa was past 40 when she founded the order for which she became famous—The Missionaries of Charity—and continued to give her life's energies to until her death at age 87. There doesn't seem to be any expiration date on doing the work of God.

As I've already stated, this book is about more than losing weight. In fact, you may not need to lose weight. If so, you are what I call a "Skinny Fat" person. You look like a skinny person, but your habits are those of a fat person. You were born with a high metabolism and probably couldn't gain weight if you tried. But even though you are skinny, it doesn't necessarily follow that you are healthy. This book is about how all of us can have the keys to a better body. It's about knowing what the Bible says about honoring God with our body. It's about how we can dedicate that body to God's service.

You probably have never seen me except in the beginning of this book. Even there you can see that I'm not a skinny guy, but I've come a long way toward having a fit body. I'm going to share with you my quest for a better body—a body that I can use to do God's will and live out His full plan for my life. I'm going to tell you the actual steps I took in acquiring a better body. I hope this book helps you do the same.

The Non-D-I-E-T Plan

In searching for an easy way to remember the four keys that make up the Bod4God plan, I began thinking of what I had discovered as a creative way to develop a body for God. I thought about the acrostic D.I.E.T as an effective way to remember the four keys. Those four keys, found in His Word (you will read the Scripture passages through this book), have helped me get to where I am now—more than 100 pounds lighter.

In the following chapters, I'm going to show you in depth what each key is and how it can work for you. This plan is not about recording every morsel of food you put in your mouth, as many diet plans insist you do; instead, it is about making better choices about what you eat. A lot of times when we think about the word "diet," we think about some crash plan or weight-loss program we've learned about and that other people say has been successful for them. You won't see me, or any of the others on this plan, measuring food. You also won't see us eating a lot of carbs or eating no carbs or eating only protein or eating no protein or living on grapefruit or bananas. The Bod4God Losing to Live plan is not a "diet" plan. It is a "live-it" plan!

I'm not following a short-term weight-loss program; I'm following a lifestyle program. I realize that only a small percentage of people who lose weight manage to keep it off. While it is wonderful to lose weight, it is more wonderful to keep it off. That's why the D.I.E.T. acrostic works so well. Because it is so easy to remember, what it represents encourages you to stay on the new course you have set for your life.

In the next few chapters, I'll go into each one of these areas in depth. You will learn how to apply each key area of D.I.E.T. to your life and make it work for you.

Self-Denial

Anorexia has never been a problem for me. Perhaps I could have been anorexic, but I'm not. Instead, as I've struggled, I've carried around more weight than God ever intended. As God began to stir in me a desire to change, I realized He needed to lead me. I asked Him to show me in His Word something that would help me build a Bod4God. I prayed, "God, give me truth from Your Word that can help me overcome this weight challenge in my life."

The passage God gave me was Matthew 16:24-25. "Then Jesus said to His disciples, 'If anyone desires to come after Me, let him deny himself, take up his cross, and follow Me. For whoever desires to save his life will lose it, but whoever loses his life for My sake will find it.'" My weight-loss program, Losing to Live, comes from this passage of Scripture. Jesus was talking to His disciples—His followers. As believers—as followers of Jesus—this passage of Scripture is addressed to me and to you. We are the "anyone" who desires to come after Him. There's more. "Let him deny himself." You see, there is no way around it. We have to deal with self. We have to learn to deny ourselves. It requires total dedication.

Dedication by Example

When Jesus was in the Garden of Gethsemane, He prayed before going to the cross. He prayed and asked the Father, "O My Father, if it is possible, let this cup pass from Me; nevertheless, not as I will, but as You will" (Matt. 26:39). The answer to the question Jesus asked the Father was that there was no other way for salvation to be achieved. There was no Plan B. It is only through His death on the cross that mankind is saved.

Jesus didn't want to die on the cross in that He didn't want to suffer the agony of crucifixion. Before He could face the crucifixion, He first had to die to self. He had to become willing to give up His life for you and me. He prayed to the Father, "Your will be done, not mine." It took dedication for Him to die on that cross for your sin and mine. He had to deny himself to achieve God's plan. He did it because there was no other way.

We, too, have to deny ourselves. We have to take up our cross. What is the cross in your life? For me, part of that cross was to give up bad eating habits and begin to exercise. If I wanted to follow Him, I had to deny myself in an area that was extremely difficult for me. So then, as much as we need to be willing to deny ourselves, even that much more do we need to be willing to follow Jesus' example by taking up our cross on a daily basis.

Live for Christ

Jesus instructed His disciples to deny themselves, take up their cross and follow Him. It is in following Him that we gain true life. When we live life for self in an attempt to "save" our life, we are sure to lose it. Trying to save our life has the attitude, "I'm going to live for myself. I'm going to do what I want to do." I had to stop doing that. I had to stop trying to save my life. I had to take up the cross of eating correctly and exercising. Losing my life was the only way I could ever hope to truly find it. And so I said, "Lord, I'm going to deny myself; I'm going to take up my eating and exercise cross and follow You. I'm going to *live* for You."

When you make the dedication—the commitment—to take up your cross, deny yourself and follow Christ, life becomes exciting. Now you can begin to discover *true* life. Jesus called it "abundant life." "The thief does not come except to steal, and to kill, and to destroy.

I have come that they may have life, and that they may have it more abundantly" (John 10:10). Sound good? Then quit trying to live for self. Begin living for Him.

My Current Lifestyle Plan

You are now on your way to developing a Bod4God lifestyle, so take a few minutes to evaluate your daily eating and exercise habits. This assessment will help you identify what "Losing to Live" really means for you.

My Current Nutritional Plan

How much water are you currently drinking each day? (Most people should drink at least eight glasses, eight ounces each, of water per day.)

Sometimes 8 / most times 3-4

Do you eat breakfast? If so, what do you eat?

Sometimes

Eggs / Bacon or Sausage

What do you eat for lunch?

vegetables

What do you eat for dinner?

Various

What do you eat for snacks?

CRACKERS - COOKIES - PICKLES - CHIPS

My Current Exercise Plan

Do you exercise at least three times a week? If so, what kind of exercise do you do? Fill in your exercise routine in the following chart.

WALKING / WEIGHTS

Sun.	NOTHING
Mon.	
Tues.	
Wed.	
Thurs.	
Fri.	
Sat.	NOTHING

A Bod4God Close-Up

Rich Kay
Lost more than 100 pounds

Before	After

On the day I tried to roll out of bed and felt the pain and extreme effort it took to do this simple thing, I got mad, and I mean *really* mad. I looked at my body and had the following self-talk:

What did you do to yourself, Rich? This is not you. Look at your old pictures. Just 10 years ago you weighed less than 200 pounds, wore 34-inch-waist jeans and felt okay to take your shirt off at the beach. Now you weigh 277 pounds and buy dark clothes to hide your fat rolls. Your waist size now exceeds your age and you are ashamed of even thinking about

going to the beach with a shirt on! It's time to change. You did not gain
this weight overnight, and it will take time to lose it.

That's how I began the journey. I started to take small steps to
change my lifestyle, and that eventually led me to lose an average of two
to four pounds a week. Some weeks I lost up to five pounds; other weeks
I would plateau and not lose any weight.

I don't think I could have lost weight if I had not become angry.
The battle of weight loss and weight maintenance is won or lost in your
head. You, too, will probably have to get mad to make the changes necessary to lose weight. Once you reach your goal, your anger will be replaced with great confidence and self-respect, and that will keep you on
track to continue the journey indefinitely.

I lost weight by doing what Pastor Steve is encouraging you to do
in this book. Make small, simple changes in the way you live and see the
rewards in weight loss and better health. Here's how I started:

- I got mad.
- I made one small, simple change to get to my goal: I parked
  the car farther from my office door.
- I recorded my beginning weight: 277 pounds.

Each week I continued my small, simple changes and added some
more, and I started to lose weight. I continued losing weight over the
next six months until I reached my six-month goal of weighing less than
200 pounds. I've lost more weight since then. I believe that if I could do
it, you can too.

I keep the weight off by continuing with a team. That has been the
biggest factor in maintaining my weight loss. I have to have team support, whether it's in print, in person or by email. I also have to keep exercising. If I go two days without sustained physical exercise, I feel it. I
call physical exercise "my little vacation." I didn't even go to the gym
until I had lost 60 pounds. Now that I go to the gym, I have to have exercise. I like pumping iron, but each person has to find his own thing
for exercise to keep going.

Now my eating habits have changed so much that when I see a chocolate chip cookie, it looks like cardboard to me. Five years ago, if you had put a Snickers candy bar and an apple on the table, I would have eaten the candy bar. Now I want the apple.

Yo-yo dieting (gaining and losing and gaining and losing weight) is not good for a body. Focus on adding good things to your diet until they crowd out the bad foods. Instead of pursuing one diet after another, I began to replace bad foods with good ones. I've done it to the point that now I've crowded out the bad foods. My kryptonite back then was Krispy Kreme donuts. I could polish off a couple of them without thinking. Now I crave the good stuff—apples, bananas, and so on.

Food is necessary. We need it to live, but we can also easily abuse it. Our bodies are basically juice extractors. We put food in, and then our bodies extract the vitamins and minerals and dump the rest.

Stay away from processed foods. The closer a food is to its source, the better it is for you. The more processed the foods you eat, the more possibilities there are for additives and calories you do not need. If your thought process is, "I'll do this for a year and see how it goes," then you'll do it for a year but it will not be a lifestyle change. On the other hand, if you can do a small, simple change for a week, you'll probably be able to maintain it. Then a snowball effect sets in. As you add more changes, you will be able to maintain them, and they will become a regular part of your life. Once your small, simple changes are locked in, bad foods will lose their appeal. You have to take stock of your successes and build on them. You have to ignore the negative thoughts that may come to your mind.

Don't beat yourself up for not losing more weight than you have, or for falling off the wagon. Failure is not final; it's feedback. Celebrate your successes. Take captive those negative thoughts and wrestle them to the ground.

We have to change how we think about food. We may think we deserve a reward of some kind, but it doesn't have to be food. I do physical exercise instead.

For me, temptation is not about sweets, but about volume—the amount of food I eat. If I can s-l-o-w down consumption of what I'm eating, I won't eat as much. For example, at parties, food might be pushed on you. Rather than gobbling it down and soon having more food pushed on you, place some food on a small salad plate, carry it around with you all evening and nurse it throughout the event.

The *T* for Team is essential to your weight loss and weight management journey. The team concept of leadership is about consistency—leading by example. What I focus on in the Losing to Live groups is accountability and communication. Get folks to talk about what's going on with them. "Where are you at now?" "It's okay. You're here. You've made a decision to change. You'll get there. Remember, 90 percent of life is showing up." Did you know that those who show up more often have the higher percentage of weight-loss success? It's because we are held to accountability at those meetings. The team is where we can find encouragement from one another.

During your journey to lose weight, focus on doing more and more small, simple changes. Surround yourself with a positive team. I did it, and you can do it too. Get some support and help from a team. *Make better choices and stay with them. Get moving. It all works together for success.*

Note: Rich Kay's book, *Small, Simple Changes to Weight Loss and Weight Management,* is available by calling 866-250-7287 or by contacting him through his website at www.SmallSimpleChanges.com.

Small Steps to Life Ideas

What Do You Need to Know About H₂O?

How did you do with drinking an adequate amount of water each day? Did you follow through with it? If yes, hooray for you! If not, try again this week. It's very important to drink water. The body is 61.8 percent water. The brain is 70 percent water. We have to have water to survive.

PHIL 3:10-14

Small Food Step

If you eat more slowly, you will consume fewer calories per meal. It takes 20 minutes for the stomach to tell the brain it's full. Train yourself to frequently put your fork down while you are eating. This gives your body an opportunity to feel satisfied before you overeat. Most of us eat so fast that we don't really taste the food. Slow down and savor each flavor. Enjoy your food, and stop eating when you're satisfied.

Small Exercise Step

Keep it simple. Just walk up the stairs rather than take the elevator. It seems like a small thing, but if a 150-pound person spends two minutes climbing the stairs, he will burn 18 calories. Want to know more? There are a number of websites where you can calculate the calories burned by the physical activities you do (a good one is http://www.health status.com/calculate/cbc).

Small Steps to Life Record

What "Skinny Things" Will You Do This Week?

Fill out this chart each week by indicating: (1) What you will do to eat less to live; (2) What you will do to exercise more to live; and (3) What average daily ounces of water you will drink. Pick only a few things and stick with them. Remember, weight loss and maintenance requires you to *eat less* and *exercise more*.

Sun.	MORE WATER / LESS JUNK / LESS FOOD LATE @ NIGHT
Mon.	
Tues.	
Wed.	
Thurs.	ZUMBA
Fri.	
Sat.	

Bod4God Victory Guide

To apply the information in this chapter to your life, work through the following Victory Guide. It will equip you to practice the four keys to weight loss. Record this week's weight change on "My Progress Report" located in appendix A. Big losers make the Victory Guide a high priority!

Week Two: Losing to Live

Memory Verse

"Then Jesus said to His disciples, 'If anyone desires to come after Me, let him deny himself, and take up his cross, and follow Me. For whoever desires to save his life will lose it, but whoever loses his life for My sake will find it'" (Matt. 16:24-25).

Reflection/Application Questions

1. In Matthew 16:24-25, Jesus stated that you must lose your life in order to live. If you want to live, you've got to deny yourself. To deny yourself means total, unconditional surrender to your Savior, Jesus Christ. In what specific ways would you need to deny yourself (surrender to Christ) to improve your health?

   CUT BACK ON SWEETS
   MORE EXERCISE

2. How have you denied yourself and allowed Jesus to be first in your life?

   CUT BACK THE SWEETS

3. If Christ is not first place in your life, what or who is?

    _____

    _____

    _____

    _____

    _____

4. Is your weight loss a "cross" in your life that you believe Jesus
    wants you to "take up"? Why do you believe it is necessary for you
    to do this? *YES!*

    MAKES ME LESS EFFECTIVE / ILLNESS

    _____

    _____

    _____

5. What are some specific things in your life that you believe God
    would want you to get rid of or deny in order to improve your
    health and lose weight?

    _____

    _____

    _____

    _____

    _____

6. What are the major principles that thread through these verses?
    Write the principles beside each verse.

    Matthew 10:39

    LIFE IS NOT IN FOOD BUT CHRIST

    _____

    _____

    _____

Matthew 16:25

THE Things of this WORLD
ARE NOT OF CHRIST

Mark 8:35

Luke 9:24

Luke 17:33

John 12:25

7. The Bible uses the word "body" 179 times. Why do you think the
   Bible says so much on this subject?

   Your body can show that you have
   no discipline.

   Your body is used for service

8. What is the difference between a weight-loss plan and a lifestyle plan?

   WEIGHTLOSS PLANS USUALLY HAVE
   AN END.

9. It will be important to have a support group to help you lose
   weight. Who are the people who will be part of your support team?
   Why did you choose each person?

My Bod4God Journal

Teach me, O Lord, the way of Your statutes, and I shall keep it to the end.
PSALM 119:33

Record what God is telling you to do this week to apply the four keys to a better body.

Dedication: Honoring God with My Body

STOP GIVING IN!

Inspiration: Motivating Myself for Change

WANT MY KIDS TO BE PROUD

Eat and Exercise: Managing My Habits

DO SOMETHING!

CUT THE SWEETS

Team: Building My Circle of Support

LOSE WEIGHT TO ENCOURAGE OTHERS.

WEEK THREE

D Is for Dedication

Walk in the Spirit, and you shall not fulfill the lust of the flesh.
GALATIANS 5:16

D is for "dedication." Dedication is important in the challenge of losing weight. We must dedicate our body to God if we are ever going to have a Bod4God.

I talk to many people each week about Losing to Live. I also do many interviews on local, national and even international radio and TV. One day a man, who was at least an agnostic, and perhaps even an atheist, asked me, "Don't you think it's possible to lose weight without God?" Theoretically, I would have to admit a person can lose weight without God. People do it all the time with secular programs. However, I knew I wasn't one of them. I couldn't lose weight without God's help. I *really* needed God to guide me in this new lifestyle.

My journey began when I dedicated myself to God. In Galatians 5:16—the Scripture at the beginning of this chapter—Paul called this concept "walking in the Spirit." As the Scripture above says, when we walk in the Spirit, we will not fulfill the "lusts of the flesh." What else could we call overeating and eating bowl after bowl of ice cream other than "fulfilling the lust of the flesh"? We have to call overeating and eating junk food what it is. We have to acknowledge what we are doing before we can begin to change. I had to bring God's Holy Spirit into my life when it came to eating and exercise. I had to depend on the Holy Spirit to guide me in my choices of food. I had to ask Him to strengthen me when it came to exercise.

The Bible says that the "flesh is weak" (Matt. 26:41). That's probably an understatement. My flesh is particularly weak when it comes to eating and exercising. The Bible also says that if you walk in the Spirit, you won't fulfill the lust of your flesh. That simply means that you will allow God's Holy Spirit to control you and your intense desires for something.

In all practicality, how does this work? I was used to letting the Holy Spirit guide me when I preached, but not when I sat down to eat. I had to learn to listen for His voice prompting me to make good choices for my body—what I ate and the amount I ate. If I truly wanted a Bod4God, I could no longer stuff whatever I craved into my mouth with wild abandon. I had to stop and think about what I was about to eat.

Many of us have a gap between our beliefs and our behavior. We know what is right, but we don't do it. James said, "Therefore, to him who knows to do good and does not do it, to him it is sin" (Jas. 4:17). I had to recognize my abusive eating for what is was—sin. I had to bring my beliefs and behavior together. For me, the first step was to dedicate my eating to God. No more playing the games of, "Well, this one bite won't hurt" or "I'll buy this treat for the kids, but I won't touch it." I had to finish with all of that. I had to learn to honor God with my body. Here is the way I approached learning to honor God with my body.

Dedicate Your Body

In Romans 12:1-2, Paul wrote, "I beseech you therefore, brethren, by the mercies of God, that you present your bodies a living sacrifice, holy, acceptable to God, which is your reasonable service. And do not be conformed to this world, but be transformed by the renewing of your mind, that you may prove what is that good and acceptable and perfect will of God." In the modern paraphrase THE MESSAGE, the concept of "dedication" is explained a little more clearly:

So here's what I want you to do, God helping you: Take your everyday, ordinary life—your sleeping, eating, going-to-work, and walking-around life—and place it before God as an offering. Embracing what God does for you is the best thing you can do for him. Don't become so well-adjusted to your culture that you fit into it without even thinking. Instead, fix your attention on God. You'll be changed from the inside out. Readily recognize what he wants from you, and quickly respond to it. Unlike the culture around you, always dragging you down to its level of immaturity, God brings the best out of you, develops well-formed maturity in you.

Paul is saying, "I am begging you earnestly, dedicate your body to God!" We are to present our bodies as "living sacrifices."

Someone once quipped that the problem with a living sacrifice is that it keeps crawling off the altar. It feels that way sometimes. We can "sacrifice" for a time, but after a while we slip up, and then we either give up or have to go back to the beginning and start again.

Sometimes, dedicating ourselves to God is as simple as just saying it. "God, I give myself to You. I give my body to You for Your purposes. I can't do this on my own. I need the help of Your Holy Spirit to remind me of my calling, to encourage me when I think I can't go on and when I think things will never change." After you pray this prayer, God will help you. He can do for you what you cannot do for yourself. He can and must empower you. He can change you from the inside out. He can renew your mind. The change He can bring is not magic, but it is miraculous.

If we are not to be conformed to the world, we have to recognize the world's view of food and eating. Eating whatever you wish seems to be considered an entitlement for the majority of the American population. You work hard, and when you come home you should be able to eat whatever you wish. You've earned it. Right?

In the United States, a large percentage of people are unhealthy because they are overweight. But no wonder. Just go to a grocery store and see how much of the food there didn't exist in its present form 20 or even 10 years ago. There are salty chips in every conceivable shape and flavor, and dozens of flavors of dips to accompany them. There are 31 (and many more) flavors of ice cream. There are sugared cereals by the trainload. There are sweetened soft drinks stacked to the ceiling. There are prime cuts of red meat laden with high-cholesterol fat. When you look at it that way, it's not a grocery store where you are shopping; it's a death trap—unless you learn to shop in a healthy way by shopping on the outside aisles of the store. That's where the living food is—the fruits, vegetables, dairy products and the like. Food on the inside aisles may have been there for months.

There is a positive side to grocery shopping as well. Once upon a time, people could only eat what was in season. Now we can get fresh fruits and vegetables all year long. We have pasteurized and fortified milk and dairy products. We can buy fresh fish and chicken all year round. We are a blessed people when it comes to grocery shopping.

If we are going to dedicate our bodies to God, we are going to have to listen to the Holy Spirit's prompting every time we approach food— and that includes when we are shopping. We cannot say, "It's my body, I can do what I want with it." If you have dedicated your body to God, then it is no longer yours. So, no, you can't do what you want with it. Philippians 3:19 talks about people "whose god is their belly." Ouch! That's harsh.

Truthfully, our belly is often all about self and doing what self wants to do. If your belly is in control of your eating and your life, you are engaging in a form of idolatry. Those of us who would never consider bowing down to a statue to worship, bow down to our appetite and make it a god. This is why the first thing I had to do to lose weight was to stop letting my belly be my god. I had to stop being an idolater. I had to admit that I had made my belly my god and then deny myself. I'm not going to pretend. It was an awful struggle; I mean really difficult.

Christians: The Most Overweight People Group in America

I said earlier that it has been determined that Christians are the most overweight people group on earth. Why is this true?

A recent survey by ChristiaNet reported that "out of 4,000 Christians surveyed, 39 percent did not feel that being overweight was sin. They believed that people were made in God's image, no matter their size: 'We are made after God's image, it doesn't matter how fat we are, He still loves us.' Some commented about the fact that God made each person unique and different: 'God didn't make everyone thin, and some people are just bigger than others.' Many in this category cited medical reasons or genetics for being overweight and that these reasons did not hold an individual responsible, 'Some people just can't help it, so you can't blame them.' "[1]

Such thinking may be one reason why being overweight is such a problem in our society, and particularly in the Christian community. You can shift the blame about being overweight to God by saying, "That's just the way He made me," but shifting the blame doesn't help you lose weight or improve your health.

Another possible reason is the lack of emphasis on health in most churches. I recently read an article about a study conducted by Ken Ferraro, Professor of Sociology at Purdue University and the Director of Purdue's Center on Aging and the Life Course, titled, "Study Finds Some Faithful Less Likely to Pass the Plate." While the reference is to the offering plate, the meaning is to Christians' propensity to overeat. In the article, Ferraro states that "religious shepherds need to keep better watch over their flocks and add activities to keep from fattening them up." He adds:

America is becoming known as a nation of gluttony and obesity, and churches are a breeding ground for this problem. . . . If religious leaders and organizations neglect this issue, they will contribute to an epidemic that will cost the health care system millions of dollars, and reduce the quality of life for many parishioners.

The reason I like this article so much is that right from the beginning Ferraro puts the blame squarely where the blame needs to go: the pastor. I believe everything rises and falls on leadership, and I believe the main reason people are overweight in the pews is because their pastors are overweight behind the pulpit.

Ferraro also concludes that Christians accept the sin of overeating. We might preach against other things, but overeating is something we don't talk about much. "Most religions also encourage restraint from participating in injurious behaviors, such as heavy drinking and smoking," Ferraro says. "However, overeating is not considered a great sin—it has become the accepted vice." Many religious activities are rooted in food, and these foods tend to be high in fat. "These high-fat meals are saying implicitly, 'This is how we celebrate,'" says Ferraro. "Instead, religious leaders need to model and encourage physical health as an important part of a person's spiritual wellbeing."

To counter these effects, Ferraro believes that churches should encourage their members to eat healthier and engage in physical activity. He suggests organized walks with the pastor after services, serving fruit and vegetables instead of heavy casseroles at church functions, and using churches' large rooms or halls for fitness classes. "With more awareness and education," Ferraro concludes, "churches can be a positive force in fighting obesity."[2]

Like many pastors, for years I chose to ignore the problem, shift blame elsewhere and not make my congregation aware of the importance of getting healthy. But not anymore. Now that I'm doing something about my weight and my lifestyle, I no longer have a difficult time speaking to my congregation about this problem, and no one can shift the blame to me for not addressing the issue. Paul said, "Therefore I testify to you this day that I am innocent of the blood of all men. For I have not shunned to declare to you the whole counsel of God" (Acts 20:26-27). Paul is saying, "Listen, my hands are clean. Your blood is not on my hands. I'm not responsible for your bad behavior. You can't blame me, because I preached to you all the counsel of God."

God tells us in His Word how to manage our bodies. That's part of the counsel of God. We've neglected this area in the Word of God. Do you know what God says to the pastors? "Take heed therefore unto yourselves, and to all the flock, over which the Holy Ghost hath made you overseers, to feed the church of God, which he hath purchased with his own blood" (Acts 20:28, KJV). We are to feed the flock, but that doesn't mean to feed the church of God potluck dinners. We've done a good job of feeding the stomachs of the people in our congregations. This verse, however, is talking about feeding their souls with the Word of God.

Once again, my answer as to why so many Christians are over-weight is because so many pastors are overweight, and those over-weight pastors have neglected this portion of the Word of God. The good news is that if the problem stands in the pulpit, perhaps the an-swer stands in the pulpit as well. If God will allow me, and I'm praying He will, I'm going to create a movement throughout this country and throughout the world that will get pastors and spiritual leaders on board with having a Bod4God and with preaching and teaching this truth to their congregations.

A Doctor Speaks

Dr. Liz Berbano is excited about the strides Capital Baptist Church is making toward physical and spiritual health. It matters to her, espe-cially because she and her husband, Darren, are medical doctors.

Liz, a former lieutenant colonel in the U.S. Army and now a staff in-ternal medicine physician at an academic medical center in Washing-ton, DC, has done her homework on weight loss. "A program will work only if there is adherence," she says. "The overriding theme to any healthy lifestyle program, as noted in several studies published recently in prominent medical journals, is that diet and exercise plans, per se, are not as important in weight loss as the motivating factors that get people to adhere to these changes."

Quoting a study in the *Journal of the American Medical Association,* Liz adds, "One way to improve dietary adherence rates . . . may be to use a broad spectrum of diet options, to better match individual patient food preferences, lifestyles, and cardiovascular risk profiles."[3] Liz be-lieves that Bod4God is seeing success because it promotes healthy eat-ing and exercise options and gives a spiritual reason for adherence that motivates spiritually minded people.

Liz is also the aerobics trainer for the church's Body & Soul fitness program (more about this program in chapter 8). The program allows participants to become physically and spiritually fit, with people en-couraging each other to stay with their healthy lifestyle changes as they bring God into this area of their lives. Students in the class exercise at various levels of intensity. Liz believes that because the program features music rich in biblical content, "'it's nourishing for the mind and heart, as well as for the body."

Once again, remember . . . weight loss begins in your head and heart. I had to realize that my body was not for the gratification of self, but for the glorification of God. God wants to be magnified in us. Paul said, "According to my earnest expectation and my hope that in nothing I shall be ashamed, but with all boldness, as always, so now also *Christ will be magnified in my body*, whether by life or by death" (Phil. 1:20, emphasis added).

To bring belief and behavior together, you need to apply dedication.

Notes

1. "Being Overweight Is Not Good," ChristiaNet. http://christiannews.christianet.com/1190131185.htm.

2. Amy Patterson Neubert, "Study Finds Some Faithful Less Likely to Pass the Plate," August 24, 2006. http://www.eurekalert.org/pub_releases/2006-08/pu-sfs082406.php.

3. M. L. Dansinger, et. al., "Comparison of the Atkins, Ornish, Weight Watchers, and Zone Diets for Weight Loss and Heart Disease Risk Reduction: A Randomized Trial," *Journal of the American Medical Association*, vol. 293, no. 1, pp. 43-53.

A Bod4God Close-Up

Diane Cornell
Lost 46 pounds

Before	After

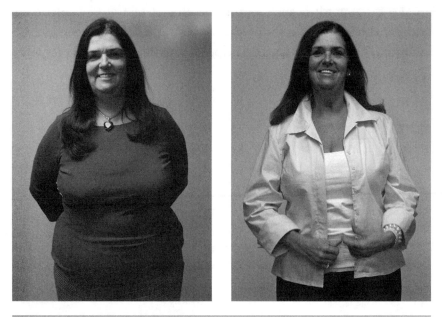

I am proud to call myself a BIG LOSER. I am a member of Capital Baptist Church and have been involved with Losing to Live since its conception. I was fortunate to be in the top five losers during the very first competition.

I joined Losing to Live in order to lose weight, but I gained *so* much more from the program. This is not like any other weight-loss program (and I know, I have been on ALL OF THEM). God made the difference for me. I have learned from my journey that God loves us and created us to have a body that is pleasing to Him, a body that is healthy and physically able to carry out the work that He has called us to do.

Bod4God has turned my life around. By dedicating my body to God, I was able to overcome the stresses in my life, which in turn helped me with my stress eating, which helped me to lose the weight. Actually, I was so involved with my daily Bible studies, memorizing Scriptures and praying for the other people on my team that the weight just fell off. A commitment to honor God with my body resulted in lasting weight loss.

God has given me the opportunity to serve as a leader in the Losing to Live program. It is such an unbelievable blessing to be able to encourage others on their journey. Being a leader has helped me be accountable for my choices and helped me grow spiritually every day. Thank you, God!

Small Steps to Life Ideas

What Do You Need to Know About H$_2$O?

Let's talk about water again because it is so vital to your weight loss. A good estimate of how much water to drink is to take your body weight in pounds and divide that number in half. That gives you the number of ounces of water per day that you need to drink. For example, if you weigh 160 pounds, you should drink at least 80 ounces of water per day. If you exercise, you should drink another eight-ounce glass of water for every 20 minutes you are active. When you are traveling on an airplane, because the pressurized air is so dry, it is good to drink eight ounces of water for every hour you are on board the plane. If you live in an arid climate, you should add another two glasses per day. As you can see, your daily need for water can add up to quite a lot.

Small Food Step

By now you have probably seen a change in your weight. If so, good for you. If you have not seen a change, and have been faithful in keeping the small steps, be patient; it will work in time. Let's add another small step to help you see the numbers on the scale move downward.

The only way anyone can lose weight is to burn up more calories than you take in. We talked about eating at a slower pace as a means of feeling full more quickly so that you can stop eating before you have eaten more than you need.

The name of the game is "portion distortion" control. A new study shows that cutting down portion size may be the single most effective thing you can do to promote lasting weight loss. Researchers found that overweight people who spent the bulk of their efforts in controlling the portion size of what they ate were more likely to lose weight and keep it off. If you are going to eat a little more of anything, make it fruit and vegetables.

Make a fist. That's about the size of your stomach. Now, be honest, if you are having weight problems, you are probably eating three or four times that much. America has become the nation of super-sized portions, and it shows in our super-sized shapes. Here are some portion sizes you need to stick to in order to lose weight:

- Meat—the size of a deck of cards
- Fish—the size of a checkbook
- Peanut butter—the size of a whole walnut
- Salad Dressing—2 tablespoons
- Butter—the size of a postage stamp
- Cereal—the size of a baseball
- Rice or pasta—the size of half a baseball
- Bread—the size of one CD
- Hard Cheese—the size of four dice
- Mixed nuts—the size of a golf ball

Small Exercise Step

Do two or three minutes of simple exercises when you first get up in the morning or go for a short walk outside. It will get your metabolism revved up, and that will help you burn calories all day. Continue to park your car a good distance from your office and take the stairs rather than the elevator.

Small Steps to Life Record

What "Skinny Things" Will You Do This Week?

Fill out this chart each week by indicating: (1) What you will do to eat less to live; (2) What you will do to exercise more to live; and (3) What average daily ounces of water you will drink. Pick only a few things, and stick with them. Remember that weight loss and maintenance requires you to *eat less* and *exercise more*.

Sun.	
Mon.	
Tues.	
Wed.	
Thurs.	
Fri.	
Sat.	

Bod4God Victory Guide

To apply the information in this chapter to your life, work through the Victory Guide. It will equip you to practice the four keys to weight loss. Big losers make the Victory Guide a high priority. Record this week's weight change on "My Progress Report" located in appendix A.

Week Three: *D* Is for Dedication

Memory Verse

"Walk in the Spirit, and you shall not fulfill the lust of the flesh" (Gal. 5:16).

Reflection/Application Questions

1. Galatians 5:16 encourages you to "walk in the Spirit," which means to allow the Holy Spirit to control you. What does God promise to you in this verse if you will walk in the Spirit?

    NOT GIVE IN TO THE FLESH

2. Is there a connection between the "lust of the flesh" and your struggle with weight? Explain.

    GOOD TASTING FOOD MAKES YOUR

    BODY FEEL GOOD.

3. Jesus said in Matthew 26:41, "The spirit indeed is willing, but the flesh is weak." How does Christ's statement represent your own Bod4God experience?

   My flesh has become stronger since the start of Bod4God.

4. In what specific ways do you need to incorporate walking in the Spirit with your eating and exercise habits?

   Do more scripture reading & keep your mind off of food

5. In Romans 12:1, Paul uses the word "sacrifice" when describing the dedication of our bodies to the Lord. What do you think you will have to sacrifice, or give up, in order to dedicate your body to God?

   Junk!

6. Philippians 3:19 talks about people "whose god is their belly." This verse teaches you that overeating can be a form of idolatry. What struggles have you had in this area? Explain.

7. As I mention in this chapter, I had to realize my body was not for the gratification of self but for the glorification of God. What does this mean to you?

_____

_____

_____

_____

_____

_____

_____

My Bod4God Journal

Teach me, O Lord, the way of Your statutes, and I shall keep it to the end.
PSALM 119:33

Record what God is telling you to do this week to apply the four keys to a better body.

Dedication: Honoring God with My Body

Keep it UP!

Inspiration: Motivating Myself for Change

LOOK AT THE RESULTS AND KNOW THAT
IT WILL ONLY GET BETTER

Eat and Exercise: Managing My Habits

STOP MAKING EXCUSES

Team: Building My Circle of Support

D Is for More Dedication

If you confess with your mouth the Lord Jesus
and believe in your heart that God has raised Him from
the dead, you will be saved.

ROMANS 10:9

Dedication requires discipline. From the time we are young we hear the word "discipline" directed toward us. When we were children, most of us didn't like the word because we thought it meant punishment—time outs, restrictions, grounding and sometimes much more. However, discipline carries a strong positive idea rather than just the negative idea we've brought from childhood. There are 11 definitions given for the word "discipline" in an online dictionary. Many of the definitions describe discipline as being the application of oneself to learning something. In fact, the most positive action definitions are: "To train by instruction and exercise; drill," and "To bring to a state of order and obedience by training and control."

In 1 Corinthians 9:27, Paul says, "But I discipline my body and bring it into subjection, lest, when I have preached to others, I myself should become disqualified." No matter what we are doing or learning to do, we must discipline our body.

Figure skaters learn the precise discipline of the required figures and spins along with complicated choreography. Competitive swimmers spend hours each day swimming back and forth in a pool, practicing the discipline of the strokes and turns while building body strength. Every sport has its disciplines. My sport was football, and I could never have played the game if I had not disciplined my body. I was on a football scholarship, and the school depended on my performance. So discipline is a good thing and something that everyone needs to practice to accomplish anything worthwhile in life.

When we talk about discipline, we are talking about something that will enhance our life and take us to a new lifestyle. In Romans 6:11-13, Paul says:

> Likewise you also, reckon yourselves to be dead indeed to sin, but alive to God in Christ Jesus our Lord. Therefore do not let sin reign in your mortal body, that you should obey it in its lusts. And do not present your members as instruments of unrighteousness to sin, but present yourselves to God as being alive from the dead, and your members *as* instruments of righteousness to God.

There's that concept again—the one about losing yourself, dying to self, being dead to sin but alive to God. The "members" referred to in this Scripture passage are our body parts. The words tell us not to yield our body parts to sin. We are rather to give those body parts (all of them) to God. I finally came to the point where I disciplined all of my body parts. It has worked for me, and now I want to invite you to join me in dedicating your body parts to God. Let's make that a little more specific by starting with your feet and work upward.

Your Feet

The Bible says that feet that are dedicated to God are beautiful: "How beautiful are the feet of those who preach the gospel of peace, who bring glad tidings of good things!" (Rom. 10:15). You need to dedicate your feet to God and say, "God, I want to be a witness for You, wherever my feet take me. Whether I go to church, to my job, to the grocery store or anywhere else, I want to be a witness for You. I'm not going to allow these feet to take me places that would displease You. I dedicate my feet to You, for Your use and for your glory."

So, how about it, friend? Will you present your feet to God right now? If so, say, "*Here are my feet, God. I give them to You for Your use.*"

Your Feet and Weight Loss:
- Use them to exercise.
- Don't use them to walk by areas of temptation. Stay out of fast-food restaurants; and stay out of the kitchen.

Your Sexuality

We are all sexual beings. God has given us sexual organs. Disciplining ourselves as instruments of righteousness to God also means disciplining our sexuality. It's important to realize that your mind is your most influential sexual organ. If you want to discipline your other sexual organs, first you need to discipline your mind. You need to pull your mind away from visual stimulation that fills it with impure sexual thoughts. You already know that there are many movies and TV shows filled with impure images and talk. Now there is the Internet and a flood of pornography that can be accessed right in your home. If we pack those evil images into our mind, we cannot assume that we will be able to discipline our mind and later on our body parts to make pure choices.

The Bible says, "For this is the will of God, your sanctification: that you should abstain from sexual immorality; that each of you should know how to possess his own vessel in sanctification and honor" (1 Thess. 4:3-4). All sex outside of marriage is sin. I'd encourage you to say out loud right here and now, "God, I'm not going to sin with my sexuality. I'm not going to get involved in fornication. I'm not going to get involved in adultery. God, I'm going to be careful about what I put into my mind so that I will not make wrong choices. Right now, I present my sexuality to You. You made sex, and you made it to be beautiful. You are pro-sex. It is the world and sin that have perverted it."

God is a cool God. He gave us sex, and when He did, He gave us some guidelines. He says that sexual activity should occur only between a husband and a wife. He said that you can have sex, but you've got to find your own husband or wife and be faithful to that person.

Even if you've made a mess of your sexuality, God will forgive you when you confess the wrong you've done and ask for His help. Are you ready to say, *"God, I present my sexuality to You"*?

Your Sexuality and Weight Loss:

- Remember to dress modestly—even after you lose weight.
- Maintain a healthy attitude toward sex.
- Remember that sex should happen only within the boundary of your marriage.

Your Emotions

We must bring our emotions under discipline. If you've ever tried a diet program before, you know that one of the first things discussed is emotional eating. Do you eat when you're stressed? When you're angry? When you're excited? One of the most detrimental emotions with regard to weight loss is bitterness. I call bitterness "frozen rage." Bitterness is a poison that can destroy your body. It is a contributing factor to many diseases. It results in depression and a feeling that life is not worth living. Your body was not designed to house bitterness. Hebrews 12:14-15 says, "Pursue peace with all people, and holiness . . . looking carefully lest anyone fall short of the grace of God; lest any root of bitterness springing up cause trouble, and by this many become defiled."

At the heart of bitterness is a lack of forgiveness. Not forgiving someone drives the issue underground where it festers and grows into a "root of bitterness." Forgiveness is not an option. It is a command: "Be kind to one another, tenderhearted, forgiving one another, even as God in Christ forgave you" (Eph. 4:32). Choose to get better and not bitter.

Perhaps even more to the point is this Scripture passage from Matthew 6:12-15: "Forgive us our debts, as we forgive our debtors. And do not lead us into temptation, but deliver us from the evil one. . . . For if you forgive men their trespasses, your heavenly Father will also forgive you. But if you do not forgive men their trespasses, neither will your Father forgive your trespasses." The cost of not forgiving others, and allowing a root of bitterness to grow inside you, is too costly to you and to your body. You must forgive, and forgive early when you have taken on an offense.

While reading this section of the book, you've had time to think about your own life and evaluate if an unforgiving attitude and a root of bitterness are affecting your ability to change your lifestyle so that you can lose weight. Are you ready to change? Are you ready to make a commitment to forgive and pull out your root of bitterness? If so, say, *"God, I want to present all my emotions to You, especially my bitter attitude."*

Your Emotions and Weight Loss:
- Keep your stress level low through prayer, exercise and reading God's Word.
- Remember that resentment only punishes you.
- Don't use food as a medication—as emotional eating.
- Remember that the Bible says, "Be anxious for nothing" (Phil. 4:6).

Your Hands

You might ask, "What do my hands have to do with losing weight?" The Bible says, "Cleanse your hands, you sinners" (Jas. 4:8). Think about what you do with your hands. I used my hands to pick up the wrong kind of food and put it in my mouth. Perhaps for you, it's not just food, but cigarettes or marijuana or many other things that are detrimental to your health and wellbeing. Perhaps it's using your hands to touch someone who is not your spouse. "Cleanse your hands, you sinners."

Let's dedicate our hands to God to do His work. Hands are an active part of our Bod4God. *"God, I'm going to honor You with my hands. I'm going to please You with my hands."*

Your Hands and Weight Loss:
- Use them to grab a bottle of water.
- Use them to detox your kitchen.
- Move them to select healthy foods and prepare healthy meals.
- Don't use them to pick up chocolate.
- Don't use them to pick up unhealthy food.

Your Mouth

The mouth (which includes the tongue) may be the most difficult body part of all to bring under discipline. I'm not talking here about what goes into your mouth as much as what comes out of it. Learning to discipline the tongue and what you say, will take you a long way toward a lifestyle change. James warned us:

> Even so the tongue is a little member and boasts great things. See how great a forest a little fire kindles! . . . But no man can tame the tongue. It is an unruly evil, full of deadly poison. With it we bless our God and Father, and with it we curse men, who have been made in the similitude of God. Out of the same mouth proceed blessing and cursing. My brethren, these things ought not to be so (Jas. 3:5,8-10).

Of course, in a book about weight loss we have to talk about disciplining ourselves concerning what we put into our mouths as well as what comes out. Proverbs 23:1-2 says, "When you sit down to eat . . . put a knife to your throat if you a man given to appetite." That's pretty severe! God doesn't actually want us to cut our throats to prevent us from overeating, but He's trying to tell us, "Hey, overeating is serious because it destroys your health." This Scripture passage is telling us to take drastic action to control overeating.

I always say, "When you love potlucks more than you love God, you have a serious problem." When "all you can eat" is the way you live, you need discipline. If you are prone to gluttony, you need to take drastic measures to bring your appetite under control. I'm a man given to appetite. Therefore, I have to take drastic measures to control what goes into my mouth.

Will you give your mouth and what comes out of it as well as what goes into it to God for His use? *"God, here's my mouth. I'm giving it to You."*

Your Mouth and Weight Loss:

- Use it to pray and ask for God's help.
- Use it to eat healthy food.
- Use it to encourage others to eat in a healthy way.
- Don't use it to speak negatively to yourself or others.

Your Eyes

King David said, "I will set nothing wicked before my eyes" (Ps. 101:3). We've already talked about movies, TV and Internet access to pornography and near-pornography that comes into our mind through our eyes. More than ever, and because of such easy access to these kinds of visual stimulation, we have to discipline our eyes. Turn off the TV. Don't go to websites that exist only to pollute your mind. Choose films wisely. Set no wicked thing before your eyes.

When we're talking television and weight loss, what about all the television advertisements for food products that do not enhance good health? There are thousands of products advertised on TV that are not healthy. Then there's the Food Channel where someone is cooking delicious-looking meals nonstop, 24/7. Yes, a few of them are promoting healthy eating, but not enough to warrant keeping the channel on all day long. We have to discipline our TV viewing.

Just a quick note to the ladies. Clothing styles get skimpier and more revealing every year. As you probably know, guys are visual. They are sexually stimulated by what they see. Can you help us out by not wearing skimpy, revealing clothing? Paul wrote to the young Timothy that women should "adorn themselves in modest apparel" (1 Tim. 2:9).

Let's all make this commitment: *"God, help me keep my eyes pure, and show me if I'm causing others to stumble in this area."*

Your Eyes and Weight Loss:

- Use your eyes to read God's Word and encourage yourself.
- Use them to read helpful information about good health.
- Use them to look in the mirror and think positive things about yourself.
- Use them to enjoy the beauty of the healthy foods God has created.
- Don't use them to watch the food channel or too much TV—get moving instead.
- Avoid the lust of the eyes, which includes focusing on unhealthy foods.

Your Ears

Let's talk about disciplining your ears. Once again, with the advent of iPods and many other ways to access audio information and music, we need a rededication of our ears to God. Keep them pure and listen to what will help you grow as a believer. James 1:19 says, "Be swift to hear, slow to speak." Above all, learn to listen with your inner ear to the voice of the Holy Spirit as He tries to guide you toward great choices that will make you a healthy person with a Bod4God.

From a weight perspective, just think about all the information about food that comes to us through our ears. We are bombarded with talk about food, not only from the media but also from any small group of people standing around chatting. Much of the time, their conversation is dominated by talking about food. We have to resist the temptation about food that comes to us through our ears.

Think about this: Eve fell into sin when she heard what the serpent said about the forbidden fruit and was encouraged to eat it. He challenged her with, "Has God indeed said, 'You shall not eat of every tree of the garden'?" (Gen. 3:1). Eve listened. She listened, she heard, she disobeyed, and she ate the fruit. Let us not listen to the temptation that comes through our ears.

Let's dedicate our ears. *"God, help me to be a listener to good things."*

Your Ears and Weight Loss:
- Use them to listen to praise music—while you exercise.
- Use them to listen to good advice from others.
- Use them to listen to God's voice.
- Use them to listen to information that will bring better health.
- Don't listen to words like "Just a little won't hurt you."

Your Mind

The Bible says, "Let this mind be in you which was also in Christ Jesus" (Phil. 2:5). That's a huge goal, and we will spend the rest of our lives striving to have the mind of Christ by surrendering our thoughts to Him in all things.

We protect our mind from evil when we discipline the rest of our body parts. If we don't allow evil to come into our mind through our eyes, ears, mouth and hands, we are protecting our mind. That's half the equation. The other half is learning how to access the mind of Christ. How would He think about certain things?

A few years ago, there was a popular campaign in the Christian community asking, "What Would Jesus Do?" It's still a valid question. One way to know how Jesus would think and act is to stop before acting and ask that question, "What *would* He do?" Of course, in order to know the answer to the question, we need to be reading the Word of God. It has all the answers for life, and it will tell us what Jesus would do in any given situation.

The standard for our thought life is Philippians 4:8:

Whatever things are true, whatever things are noble, whatever things are just, whatever things are pure, whatever things are lovely, whatever things are of good report, if there is any virtue and if there is anything praiseworthy—meditate on these things.

Make a new commitment to discipline your mind. Say, "God, take my mind and set it on things that bring You glory."

Your Mind and Weight Loss:
- Think about God.
- Allow Christ to renew your mind on a daily basis.
- Use your mind to research and gather new information on health.
- Think about what you are eating.

Your Heart

Last of all, discipline your heart. Just how do you do that? Romans 10:9 says, "If you confess with your mouth the Lord Jesus and believe in your heart that God has raised Him from the dead, you will be saved." First, you have to dedicate your heart to God through forming a relationship with him. You have to become a follower of Jesus Christ. The way to do this is to realize you are a sinner and have broken God's laws. The Bible says that because we have broken His laws, we deserve eternal death and hell. But Jesus, the sinless Son of God, came to earth, died on the cross for our sins, was buried and rose from the grave to give us eternal life through Him. To be forgiven and have eternal life we must follow the formula in Romans 10:9 above. Confess and believe, and you will be saved. It's so simple that many people miss it.

Discipline comes when we make sure that what our lips say and our heart believes are the same. Jesus talked about people who honor Him with their lips, but their hearts are far from Him. If you have never confessed Jesus Christ as your Lord and Savior and come to believe in Him as the only one who can save you from both the penalty and the power of sin, then your lips and your heart are in two different places. Here's the way to make the commitment to bring them together:

Dear God, I'm a sinner. Because of my sin, I deserve to spend eternity in hell. I believe Jesus died on the cross, was buried and rose from the grave for my sins. I turn from my sins and put my faith in Jesus Christ to get me to heaven. Thank You for saving me today, and help me to serve You the rest of my life. In Jesus' name I pray. Amen.

Your Heart and Weight Loss:
- Accept Jesus Christ as your Savior and Lord.
- Don't let a root of bitterness grow in you, cultivate a heart of forgiveness toward others.
- Love God with all your heart.

A Bod4God Close-Up

Eric Larsen
Lost more than 100 pounds

Before **After**

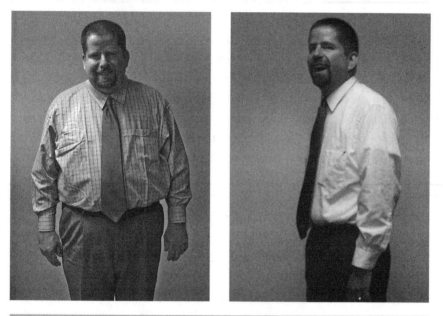

I had been overweight since I was 13 years old. I used to eat all the leftovers from my sisters' plates. I'd always had a big stomach, and kids picked on me and called me names, but I didn't care. At 25, I moved out of my parents' house. I had been sedentary before, but then it got even worse. People told me I needed to lose weight. I knew it was true, but I wasn't willing to change. Then, two years ago, I realized that I had a big problem. My clothing just got bigger and bigger. I had sleep apnea and borderline cholesterol problems. I was addicted to diet soft drinks. At the time, I worked in a restaurant. There are studies that show how working in a food establishment adds to a person's weight problems. I had the worst eating problems you could imagine.

Then I decided to join the Losing to Live competition. In the beginning, I used Slimfast to help me get started. I prayed that God would give me a taste for fruits and vegetables. Before He answered my prayer, I hardly ever ate a fruit or vegetable. God did answer my prayer, and the way it happened was at the luncheon held on the first day of the kickoff for the Losing to Live competition. A chef in our church prepared the noon meal. The meal was a healthy selection of salads and wraps, and every dish was delicious.

I have always been a meat and potatoes man, but the chef served a green bean salad, and I found out that vegetables can be delicious. Now I eat broccoli, apples, carrots and bananas every day. For dessert I eat graham crackers and a banana or an apple or strawberries. I base my diet on The Mayo Clinic's pyramid. I eat two servings of meat a day; and once a week, one of those meats is fish or tuna. Other meats I eat are chicken, a little pork and occasionally turkey sausage. I rarely eat white bread.

I also have a "cheat" day. On that day I eat some of the things I used to eat, but now I eat them in a limited way. I may not set aside a whole day for eating what I want. It might just be a day or an evening meal. If I ever have chocolate, I eat it on my cheat day or at a cheat meal.

I used to drink six diet soft drinks a day. I went off drinking diet sodas cold turkey and started drinking water. Now I drink all the water I am supposed to drink. I exercise by walking and jogging, and I participated in the Losing to Live 5K walk/run. My high cholesterol is now in the normal range. I now maintain my body to prevent illness just like you would maintain a car to prevent mechanical problems.

As far as inspiration goes, Pastor Steve has been my main inspiration. I'm now a team captain and I'm inspiring others to make healthy changes in their lives. I had one of the top 10 losers on my team in the last competition. It is amazing that others are looking to me for inspiration. I know it would be easy to gain the weight back. But I'm motivated by my desire to be faithful and accountable to the team, and because I don't want to have to buy a whole new wardrobe!

Small Steps to Life Ideas

What Do You Need to Know About H_2O?

In addition to making healthy nutritional choices and exercising daily, drinking adequate amounts of water is also extremely beneficial for weight loss. Avoiding dehydration is crucial if you are trying to lose weight. This is true for several reasons, but one of the most pertinent factors has to do with water's effect on the body's vital organs. Studies have shown that a low consumption of water allows more fat to be deposited instead of being metabolized into energy. Water helps our kidneys to flush out toxins. The kidneys cannot perform their function properly without water, and this forces the liver to assist with water filtration. The result is interference in the liver's primary function, which is to burn fat. So drink a sufficient amount of water!

Small Food Step

Nobody can keep to a totally restrictive diet that never allows a treat. Just make sure that your "treats" are healthy, such as fat-free yogurt sprinkled with a few nuts; strawberries dipped in a tiny bit of melted dark chocolate; a cup of melon pieces; a few pretzels—not the whole bag.

Small Exercise Step

Anyone can find 30 minutes a day for exercise. Here are some ways:

- Give up one TV sitcom rerun and exercise instead. Or get a treadmill and walk on it while you watch TV.
- Walk while listening to books on tape or on an iPod. It will make your walk time seem shorter.
- Walk to errands or appointments rather than take the car.
- Work around your house—indoors or out. Housework and gardening can burn quite a number of calories.

- Chase a kid. Baby-sit for a young mother or a single parent who needs a break. It helps you and it helps them. Toddlers never sit still, so you'll have to chase them around to keep them out of trouble.
- Get a dog and walk it.

Small Steps to Life Record

What "Skinny Things" Will You Do this Week?

Fill out this chart each week by indicating: (1) What you will do to eat less to live; (2) What you will do to exercise more to live; and (3) What average daily ounces of water you will drink. Pick only a few things, and stick with them. Remember that weight loss and maintenance requires you to *eat less* and *exercise more*.

Sun.	
Mon.	
Tues.	
Wed.	
Thurs.	
Fri.	
Sat.	

Bod4God Victory Guide

To apply the information in this chapter to your life, work through the Victory Guide. It will equip you to practice the four keys to weight loss. Big losers make the Victory Guide a high priority. Record this week's weight change on "My Progress Report" located in appendix A.

Week Four: *D* Is for More Dedication

Memory Verse

"If you confess with your mouth the Lord Jesus and believe in your heart that God has raised Him from the dead, you will be saved" (Rom. 10:9).

Reflection/Application Questions

1. How would you state this week's memory verse, Romans 10:9, in your own words?

   _____

   _____

   _____

   _____

   _____

   _____

   _____

2. Has there ever been a time when you dedicated your heart and life to Jesus Christ? Describe this event and the way it changed the way you live.

   _____

   _____

   _____

   _____

   _____

   _____

   _____

3. Take some time to think about your body and your health while the information you have just read is still fresh in your mind. What steps do you plan to take to change each part of your body? List these in the chart below.

Body Area	What steps do you need to take in relationship to your health to dedicate each area to God?
Feet	
Sexuality	
Emotions	
Hands	
Mouth	
Eyes	
Ears	
Mind	
Heart	

4. Within the context of weight loss, which of your body members are most difficult to discipline?

_____

_____

_____

_____

_____

_____

5. Why do you think this area is such a struggle for you?

_____

_____

_____

_____

_____

_____

6. The title of this book, *Bod4God,* is used throughout the text. Now that you have completed this part of the study, what does the term "Bod4God" mean to you?

_____

_____

_____

_____

_____

_____

_____

_____

My Bod4God Journal

Teach me, O Lord, the way of Your statutes, and I shall keep it to the end.
PSALM 119:33

Record what God is telling you to do this week to apply the four keys to a better body.

Dedication: Honoring God with My Body

_____
_____
_____
_____
_____

Inspiration: Motivating Myself for Change

_____
_____
_____
_____
_____

Eat and Exercise: Managing My Habits

_____
_____
_____
_____

Team: Building My Circle of Support

_____
_____
_____
_____
_____

I Is for Inspiration

The thief does not come except to steal, and to kill, and to destroy. I have come that they may have life, and that they may have it more abundantly.

JOHN 10:10

Most of us know that we need to get healthier. The problem is that we're not motivated to do anything about it other than talk about it; and once in a while we get started and then give up within a week or two when we are not satisfied with the results. In this chapter, we're going to talk about how to get motivated and stay that way. Weight loss is about a lifestyle change, and it won't happen unless you are inspired to take those first steps and then stay with the program.

Some of us become inspired when the doctor tells us that if we don't lose weight we're going to lose our life. Some of us get sick of not being able to tie our shoes without huffing and puffing over a big stomach. Some of us have an event to attend for which we want to lose weight. It doesn't matter what the inspiration is, the important part is to find out what works for you and get going on a plan.

To encourage you, let me remind you that by making Small Steps to Life in your diet and exercise routine, you can begin to reduce your waistline. It isn't complicated. It isn't costly. But it does take determination and commitment, and lots of it.

Your Body Was Created for God

Let me remind you once again that your first inspiration must be to remember that your body was created by God and for Him. God gave you life. God sustains your life. God is the one keeping your heart beating and your brain functioning.

God cares about our bodies. He cares if we are healthy or not. I believe this, and it's why my church and I are on the front lines of the fat fight. It's also one of the reasons the media is so interested in what we are doing. It's a new concept to many people that God cares about our health. Many journalists who interview me are merely looking at the physical side of things. This fight, however, is also a spiritual battle. The enemy of our souls is as interested in us being overweight, without energy and unhealthy as God is in us being at the right weight, having energy and becoming healthy. We are not going to be our most effective in God's kingdom if we cannot function at peak physical efficiency.

Where Can We Find Inspiration?

The first question of the Westminster Shorter Catechism confession of faith is: "What is the chief end of man?" The answer is: "To glorify God and enjoy Him forever." If we are to glorify God, can we do it with a body given over to gluttony? Can we glorify Him with a body that we've failed to consider is His abode on earth? So how do we come to the place where we are inspired to face this giant of a challenge in our life and begin to take steps to slay it so that we can glorify God and enjoy Him forever?

In a joyous burst of enthusiasm, the apostle Paul writes, "Now may the God of hope fill you with all joy and peace in believing, that you may abound in hope by the power of the Holy Spirit" (Rom. 15:13). And the writer of Hebrews declares with great joy, "[Look] unto Jesus, the author and finisher of our faith, who for the joy that was set before Him endured the cross, despising the shame, and has sat down at the right hand of the throne of God" (Heb. 12:2).

The Bible contains the inspiration we need for all of the challenges of life, including the challenge of losing weight. For me, Matthew 16:24-25, with regard to denying myself, taking up my cross and following Jesus, was a huge inspiration for change. I had to realize that life wasn't going to be easy as I began to deny myself. I was going to have to lose a favorite part of my life—eating lots of food. Then I began to realize that giving up the overindulgence of food was the only way for me to find my life. That was very exciting!

God gave me the verses in Matthew 16:24-25 to encourage me. I knew I wanted to experience the fullness of life in Christ. I wanted to be a fit tool for His use. I wanted to be well and happy and live to see my grandchildren and maybe even my great-grandchildren. I wanted to find my life, and here in this verse, I found out how to do it—deny myself, take up my cross, and follow Him.

Simple . . . and very difficult to do. But there's good news on that front. The Bible says, "I can do all things through Christ who strengthens me." (Phil. 4:13). Christ is so prolife that when you set out to do something difficult like getting a Bod4God, He's right there to help you live.

There's a war going on between the Lord Jesus and Satan over you and your body. Satan doesn't want you to succeed in weight loss or anything else that will make you more effective for God. Satan is a thief who will rob you of good health. He'll do everything he can to discourage you. In John 10:10, Jesus says, "The thief does not come except to steal, and to kill, and to destroy." But there's good news in the rest of the verse. Jesus says, "I have come that they may have life, and that they may have it more abundantly."

"Abundant" isn't a word we use too often these days, but we should use it when we are talking about God's goodness and grace and His ability to help us. The dictionary definitions of the word "abundant" will bless your soul. It means, "present in great quantity; more than adequate; over-sufficient, well supplied, richly supplied." He's got everything you need to give you a new life—one that works for Him, one that is able to do His will, one that is eternal.

I realized the thief was coming into my life through too much food and too little exercise. Satan was stealing from me. I had diabetes, and diabetes can kill you. Satan was killing me with a knife and fork, and I wanted to live. I wanted to receive the promise Jesus gave—the promise of life more abundantly. What I wanted was a better quality of life and a better quantity of life. I had to lose myself so that I could live. That's what inspired me—the desire to live.

Be Inspired to Leave a Legacy
of Health to Your Children

Young people need the guidance of their parents. I want to be on earth
as long as I can to be an influence in my children's lives. I want to see my
grandchildren and I want them to see me eating a healthy diet, exercising and taking care of my body. I want to be a good example to them.

I don't know how anyone could love his or her children more than
I love mine. My three kids are now young adults. Crystal, Sarah and Jeremiah are all precious to me. I don't know what might happen with
Capital Baptist Church in the future. I don't know what my legacy will
be at the church. That's up to God. I am most concerned, however,
about the legacy I am leaving my children, and I want it to be a positive
one. What am I teaching them about food and dedication and discipline and denial? What kind of example am I setting for them? In the
past I did not set a good example for them. I was not leaving them a
legacy of health. But now, I can answer the question positively, knowing that I've taken the steps needed to have a Bod4God.

Mike Huckabee, former governor of the state of Arkansas, and talk
show host, doesn't know it, but he's on my team. He lost more than 100
pounds and wrote a book called *Quit Digging Your Grave with a Knife and
Fork*. That's a book you need to own even if you only look at the cover
once in a while. That cover, that title, can be an inspiration in your
struggle to keep on track. It was after I read the book that I lost weight
and went from being diabetic to being free of diabetes. Still today, every
time I look at Huckabee's book, I am reminded that I want to live. I
want to leave that legacy of good health to my children. I want to be
around to enjoy old age with my wife.

Be Inspired to Give a Good Account to God

One day we are all going to stand before God and give an account of
our lives. Romans 14:10-12 says, "But why do you judge your brother?
Or why do you show contempt for your brother? For we shall all stand
before the judgment seat of Christ. For it is written: 'As I live, says the
LORD, every knee shall bow to Me, and every tongue shall confess to

God.' So then each of us shall give account of himself to God."

The big things for which we'll give an account include:

- Our *time*. We all have the same amount of time (24 hours in a day), and we're going to have to answer God for how we used our time.
- Our *talents*. What did we do with the talents God gave us?
- Our *treasure*. We'll have to answer God about our money and how we used it.
- Our *temple*, what we did with our body. One day you are going to deliver your body to God and say, "God, here I am, standing in judgment before You." God's going to shine His light on our time, talents and treasure, and He will also look at our temple.

In 2 Corinthians 5:10, Paul writes, "For we must all appear before the judgment seat of Christ, that each one may receive the things done in the body, according to what he has done, whether good or bad." Will you be able to give a good account to God?

An Inspiring Story of Overcoming Addiction

If you eat more than your body needs, you are addicted to food. A few years ago, a wonderful story was told in the Condensed Book section of a *Reader's Digest* magazine about a Baptist pastor. His name was Gordon Weekley, and he was in a hurry to build his church and congregation in his church-planting endeavor. His people responded to his inspiring messages as they, along with Gordon, envisioned what their church would be like.

Soon the church needed two Sunday morning services. He became busier and busier, and his wife only saw him at bedtime, and his children even less. On a visit to his physician, he explained that while life was going well, he sometimes felt a little jittery. Weekley was having trouble falling asleep once he finally crawled into bed. The doctor prescribed something to "help him sleep."

It worked and he slept deeply and woke refreshed until a little later in the day when the anxiousness returned. He didn't worry, as he knew he would sleep that night. Then the pills didn't work so well and he began to take one-and-a-half and then two. He stopped eating supper thinking that maybe the pills would work better on an empty stomach. He started losing weight.

Along the way, he started taking another drug to help him feel peppier after having taken the drugs that made him able to sleep. He was glad for the extra energy as he cared so much about his church and his people. He wanted to be everywhere at once and he didn't know if it was because he loved them or because he wanted to be loved.

Finally, his physician realized just how many prescriptions his office was writing for him and told Gordon to go get checked out at the hospital. Gordon went willingly, all the while saying, "I can stop taking the pills any time I want." But he couldn't and his life spiraled downward rather quickly.

It was his wife who first tried to call him to accountability, but he would have none of it. His denial was so deep that he could not admit that he was a drug addict, and without that admission, nothing could change. Finally, his wife had had enough. She packed her bags, took his four sons and left. He went to his study and wrote a letter of resignation from the church he'd worked so hard to build.

Life went from bad to much worse as he wandered from family member to family member and then on to friends and finally to wandering the streets in a drug-induced stupor. At last, a friend called on the phone and confronted him. "Gordon, this thing has been going on a long time. You've tried everything, and nothing has worked. I think there is one thing you haven't tried. You haven't tried God."

Of course, Gordon denied this vehemently. He said that he had prayed and asked God for help—over and over again.

"But," his friend persisted, "have you ever really, truly, given this over to Him? Recommit yourself. Pray with me now."

His friend prayed for this poor lost man and asked God to return him to the fold. Gordon hung up the phone, went to his bedroom and went down on his knees. There, he admitted that he couldn't handle his own life anymore and that he wasn't getting better. He put himself in God's hands, and then rose and went to bed. He fell asleep knowing that he had come to the end of himself and couldn't "fix" it this time. It was out of his hands.

Gordon didn't see any visions that night—he just went to sleep—and in the morning, he opened his eyes and saw only the ceiling of his bedroom. Something had changed in him, however: he felt no anxiety. He knew that he would be facing another day without pills, but he suddenly felt no desire for them. He felt calm, refreshed and at peace.

It's so utterly simple, Gordon thought. *I've preached it over and over, and I still didn't see it. "Put yourself in God's hands." How could I have missed it all these years?*[1]

That was the miraculous end of Gordon Weekley's terrible addiction. While we may not believe that our addiction is as serious as his, it might well be. God is available to deliver you from your food addiction in the same way he delivered Gordon. Think hard about the way in which Gordon Weekley stopped denying that he had a problem, put himself in God's hands and then rose and went to bed. He rested in God's ability to do the work in his life that he could not do. That same power is available to deliver you.

Note

1. Don Jeffries, "Pastor, Father, Addict," *Reader's Digest* condensed book, June 1992.

A Bod4God Close-Up

Ray Raysor
Lost 53 pounds

Before   **After**

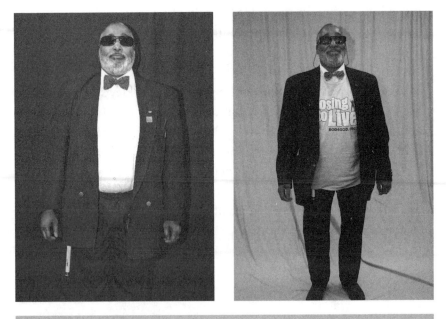

The Losing to Live 5K Walk/Run sizzled with excitement. As groups formed, I formed a "pair" with my seeing-eye dog, Rayna. Let's be clear. I'm blind. I'm not "visually impaired" or "sight challenged" or any other politically correct language. I'm blind.

I make my living as a food contractor for the federal government. I also operate a deli, a café and a gift shop. Pastor Steve challenged me that if my food was that good, how could I be the biggest loser?

When my doctor told me I was a borderline diabetic, it sobered me up. A side effect of diabetes is losing the sensation in the fingertips.

This could affect my ability to read Braille or play the piano—and my diabetes was preventable! I had hoped one day to go to the mission field and teach cane travel and the abacus to the blind in other countries. Now, all that was in jeopardy. I had chosen a season of pleasure resulting in a lifetime of diminishing health. Something had to change.

When my doctor told my wife that I—a meat eater—needed to change my eating habits to include grains, vegetables and limited fruits, my wife asked if we could start it the following week instead of immediately. The doctor was puzzled. My wife said, "First, I have to tell him what vegetables are and then I have to get him to eat them."

In spite of the doctor's dire warning, I still couldn't diet on my own. I knew I needed a team—an accountability partner. Then I heard about the Losing to Live competition from a radio advertisement. My wife and I went to check out the program and I signed up.

My exercise regimen and eating patterns changed dramatically. I knew I had to make a lifestyle change. Sure, I wanted to relapse to old behaviors. I knew that food would be a constant challenge in my line of work. Now, however, I have the tools that I built week by week during the competition instead of a only having a quick-fix solution. I still work with food, but now instead of gorging on it, I just sample it to make sure it tastes good.

Rayna, my beloved seeing-eye dog, contracted cancer and died suddenly. I am training to get another dog. As the biggest loser in the fifth competition, I am looking forward to the next competition. Hopefully, I'll have my new dog by then. Look for us in the next 5K! I'm excited because my new Bod4God will allow me to one day achieve my goal of going to the mission field. Bod4God and the Losing to Life competition have changed my life.

Small Steps to Life Ideas

How are you doing? Have you memorized any of the weekly Bible verses? If you have, you can meditate on them when temptation comes calling and when it just seems too hard to go on. That's important, so keep trying to memorize a verse a week. Now for some more small steps to add to those that have worked successfully for you.

What Do You Need to Know About H₂O?

We are still talking about water because it is so important. Did you know that if you have a mere two-percent drop in the body's water supply, it can trigger fuzzy short-term memory, trouble with basic math and difficulty focusing on smaller print such as that on a computer screen? Mild dehydration is one of the most common causes of fatigue. For the most part, the majority of the population is going around somewhat dehydrated, and this is in a country where all we have to do is turn on a tap for clean water. It doesn't make sense, does it?

Small Food Steps

Detoxify your kitchen. If you haven't done so yet, go through your cupboards and refrigerator and get rid of every snack and food that is unhealthy. There are those of us who cannot have food items like ice cream, peanut butter, packages of cookies, chips and . . . you know where your weakness is. Dump it—and don't go dig it out of the garbage later when you're hungry. It's a simple fact that if you don't have junk food in your house, you are much less likely to eat it.

Small Exercise Steps

If you like riding a bicycle, do it now. It's a great way to develop muscle, burn fat, work your heart and get that metabolism up. Oh, and it can be a lot of fun too. And then, if you're out in the sunshine, you're soaking up that vitamin that suddenly everyone is talking about and recommending—vitamin D. Don't forget to wear a helmet and keep to safe bike paths.

If you have a bike but aren't ready to get outside and ride in front of everyone, you can get a bike stand that turns your bike into an exercise machine. You can use it at home for all the same benefits and watch TV while you're exercising. Bike stands cost from $75 to $100. That's a lot cheaper than joining a club.

Small Steps to Life Record

What "Skinny Things" Will You Do this Week?

Fill out this chart each week by indicating: (1) What you will do to eat less to live; (2) What you will do to exercise more to live; and (3) What average daily ounces of water you will drink. Pick only a few things, and stick with them. Remember that weight loss and maintenance requires you to *eat less* and *exercise more*.

Sun.	
Mon.	
Tues.	
Wed.	
Thurs.	
Fri.	
Sat.	

Bod4God Victory Guide

To apply the information in this chapter to your life, work through the Victory Guide. It will equip you to practice the four keys to weight loss. Big losers make the Victory Guide a high priority. Record this week's weight change on "My Progress Report" located in appendix A.

Week Five: *I* Is for Inspiration

Memory Verse

"The thief does not come except to steal, and to kill, and to destroy. I have come that they may have life, and that they may have it more abundantly" (John 10:10).

Reflection/Application Questions

1. In John 10:10, John tells us that Satan wants to destroy us. He steals from us and attacks us during our weakest moments and in our weakest areas. When you examine your own health issues regarding weight, where does Satan attack you, and what is he stealing from you?

   Spirit of LAZINESS

2. When Jesus states that He came to give you an abundant life, this includes your health. What part of your health/weight do you think the Holy Spirit would have you change to live abundantly?

   MORE EXERCISE

3. You will have to give an account to God for how you use your time, talents, treasure and temple. What specific things do you need to do now to prepare for this final judgment?

Share the Gospel more

4. In Matthew 21:12, Jesus got mad and drove out the greedy money changers out of the Temple because they were not respecting it. In a similar way, 1 Corinthians 6:19 states that your body is the temple of the Holy Spirit. Are you mad at Satan's influence over your eating and exercise habits and the negative impact it is having on you health? Explain your answer.

I'm mad at MYSELF!

5. Look up the following verses. How could each verse motivate you when the going gets rough?

Proverbs 16:3 _Focus on God & His Spirit_
& HE will guide your steps

Jeremiah 32:27

It CAN be done!

Romans 6:6-7

Move on from my old ways
AND habits

1 Corinthians 6:12

Don't give in just because
I CAN.

Ephesians 6:11

Use every tool Available to me.

Philippians 3:13-14

Hang in there, It may take awhile, but it will happen.

6. There is power in God's Word. Do you have a Bible verse that you have claimed for maintaining a Bod4God lifestyle? If so, what is it? If not, find a verse that you can claim for your victories and recite when temptation surrounds you. Write the verse below.

1 COR 6:19 = Or do you not know that your body is the temple of the Holy Spirit who is in you, whom you have from God, and you are not your own?

JAMES 4:17 = To him who knows to do good and doesn't do it, to him is sin!

7. What is your motivation for losing weight?

GOD - FAMILY - HEALTH - APPEARANCE

My Bod4God Journal

Teach me, O Lord, the way of Your statutes, and I shall keep it to the end.
PSALM 119:33

Record what God is telling you to do this week to apply the four keys to a better body.

Dedication: Honoring God with My Body

_____
_____
_____
_____
_____

Inspiration: Motivating Myself for Change

_____
_____
_____
_____

Eat and Exercise: Managing My Habits

_____
_____
_____
_____

Team: Building My Circle of Support

_____
_____
_____
_____

I Is for More Inspiration

I can do all things through Christ who strengthens me.
PHILIPPIANS 4:13

One huge reason why people set out to lose weight but fail is because they have unrealistic goals for weight loss. Of course, magazines and television, weight-loss camps and a host of other unrealistic information causes us to believe that you set out to lose weight and it just falls off. You've probably discovered it's not true. And when we don't reach the unrealistic goals we've set, we become discouraged and reach for the chips and dip to dull our discouragement.

We have to get real. Even if we lose weight, most of us are not going to look like the models in magazines or even the people in weight-loss ads. First of all, those images have probably been computer enhanced and you wouldn't recognize the models if you met them on the street. So let's set some realistic goals about how we will look when we lose weight. We have to learn to accept our bodies. When you lose weight, you won't suddenly have blue eyes and curly hair—unless you had them before you lost weight. You probably won't have fabulous six-pack abs even if you exercise a lot. But you will look better than you do in your overweight condition, and you will definitely feel better. So get real about what losing weight is going to do for you.

Here are some things to keep in mind when you are trying to reach a weight goal:

- Action drives motivation.

- If you step on the scale and see no weight loss (or perhaps only a little) remember that it took you a while to gain all this weight and it will take you time to lose it. It will happen if you stick to your goal of creating a Bod4God lifestyle.

- Take a look back and see how far you've already come. And remember that even if you are not losing weight this week, if you're not gaining any, you are making progress.

- If you miss exercise one day, or eat something you know will not help you reach your goal, get back on track the next day or the next time you eat.

- Spend a few minutes remembering that a worthwhile payoff lies ahead. You will be an improved you.

- Remember all the benefits of exercise over and above weight loss: such as the fact it improves mood, combats chronic disease, helps manage weight, strengthens the heart and lungs, and promotes better sleep.

Setting Goals

Someone once said that if you don't set a goal, how will you know where you are going and how will you know when you arrive? And when you get back, how will you know where you've been? It is important to set goals and it is important to keep that goal in front of you. Write down your weight loss goal on a sticky note and post it on your bathroom mirror. Post it in the front of this book. Post it on a computer screen or on the dashboard of your car.

Setting a goal tends to focus you on what you want to achieve. It's like a contract with yourself. It drives your motivation. Keep the goal achievable. Set your goals realistically so that you can be successful. That will keep you motivated. Here are some tips for goal setting:

- Write down your goal. Post it where you see it often.

- Make the goal attainable. "I will lose one to two pounds a week."

- Let everyone know about your goals and get people to encourage you. Spouses and children are notorious for trashing weight-loss plans. Explain to them what you are trying to achieve, a Bod4God, and ask them to be supportive.

- Vary your exercise and try to have fun. Take a walk one day, lift weights the next, ride a bike, swim or play basketball or handball. Watching TV while moving your body can help take the tediousness out of exercise and give you something to look forward to during that time.

- Try new seasonings and flavors in your food but stay away from any that add calories. There are tons of recipes online for healthy, delicious dishes that will bring new flavors to your palate. Type the words "weight loss recipes" into an Internet search engine for more healthy food ideas than you will live long enough to eat. The Mayo Clinic has a great website for recipes. I also like the recipes at firstplace4health.com.

- Reward your success on reaching your goal, but don't do it with food. This is one of the toughest places to retrain yourself, because most of us have been rewarded with food from the time we were sitting in a highchair.

- Remember the Scripture, "I can do all things through Christ who strengthens me" (Phil. 4:13).

Four Spiritual Motivators for Change

1. Rely on God

The number-one way for me to stay motivated is to rely on God. There is no way I could have achieved my goals without the help of the Lord. When I rely on Him, I am not alone. He is with me. As I've already said, I have had a lot of people contact me about my weight loss and about our Losing to Live Weight Loss Competition. I've made it a priority to talk to them because I wanted to learn what was going on in their lives.

I try to connect what is happening in their lives with the culture in which they live. I want to know others' struggles so that I can make this message practical and relevant to readers.

When Jesus' disciples fell asleep in the Garden of Gethsemane rather than staying awake with Him to pray, Jesus said to them, "Watch and pray, lest you enter into temptation. The spirit indeed is willing, but the flesh is weak" (Matt. 26:41). That admonition was not just for those sleepy disciples, it's for all of us who seek to improve our bodies for God's use by losing weight. Even though I knew for a long time that I needed to get healthy and needed to lose weight and exercise, my spirit was willing, but my body wouldn't cooperate. One of the functions of the Holy Spirit is as a helper. I had to learn to pray specifically for the power of the Holy Spirit to fill my life and help me. I had to learn to walk in the Spirit—at the dinner table, in my recliner after dinner and at church functions where there was an overabundance of food. I made a conscious decision to walk in the Spirit on those occasions. What went for the eating part of the equation also went for the exercise part. The Holy Spirit had to help me get moving. I literally had to "move" with the Holy Spirit.

2. Refine Your Attitude

One of the first things I had to do in achieving a Bod4God was to re-fine my attitude. The Bible says, "As he thinks in his heart, so is he" (Prov. 23:7). In other words, "Your attitude, not your aptitude, deter-mines your altitude in life." I had some unhealthy attitudes to work through before I could rise above my weight, and perhaps you do too.

Do you reject your body? Some of us look at our bodies and say, "God, You messed up when You made me." Most overweight people suffer from low self-esteem. For some people it starts in childhood when they are presented with Ken and Barbie dolls. I decided that my girls were not going to have Barbie dolls. I didn't want them picking up the perfect body, no acne, impossible-to-achieve looks and shape as a model for what they should look like when grown. My son didn't have Ken or G. I. Joe dolls, either. Those male counterparts to Barbie are as ridiculously unachievable as are the female dolls. I certainly have never looked like either Ken or G. I. Joe. When I was growing up, I looked more like Mr. Potato Head or the Pillsbury Dough Boy.

With regard to the body that God gave you, the important thing to remember is that He gave it to you. And no matter how much you try to change it through weight loss or surgery or exercise, you are still stuck with the basic framework you got when you were born. The best thing you can do is to learn to love your body, treat it well and realize that while it's not perfect, it is the temple of God.

The key here is balance. We are to love and care for our body, but not make it an idol that consumes our thinking and our time. Remember, God says that we are "fearfully and wonderfully made" (Ps. 139:14).

3. Read the Bible Every Day

I can't emphasize enough that the Bible is the recorded Word of God given to us. It is a "living word" that brings health and vitality to our inward life. It's the way we renew our minds. It's the way we get to know the Author and His Son. It provides the encouragement to put off our former lifestyle and take up a new one. Ephesians 4:23 says, "Be renewed in the spirit of your mind." That's it. Feed your mind with healthy thoughts just as you feed your body with healthy food.

In addition to reading the Bible, meditate on it. Think about what you are reading. When you were little, your mother told you to chew your food thoroughly. (That's still good advice for weight loss. It helps you feel satisfied with less food.) The same goes for God's Word. Chew on it. Extract the meaning. Apply what you read to your own life. Make decisions based on what you've read and learned.

Joshua gave this instruction to God's people: "This Book of the Law shall not depart from your mouth, but you shall meditate in it day and night, that you may observe to do according to all that is written in it. For then you will make your way prosperous, and then you will have good success" (Josh. 1:8).

4. Read Health-Related Books or Materials Every Day

There are thousands of books and magazines on health, diet and exercise. I'm a busy guy and I don't have time to read lots and lots of stuff.

But every day I try to read some kind of health-related materials to feed my mind a little bit and get me thinking about what I need to be thinking about. We have a model in Paul. In 2 Timothy 4:13, Paul asked Timothy to, "Bring the cloak that I left with Carpus at Troas when you come—*and the books, especially the parchments*" (emphasis added). The parchments were the Word of God, but it appears that Paul had an interest in other kinds of good books.

Hosea 4:6 says, "My people are destroyed for lack of knowledge." Today there is no excuse for anyone to have a lack of knowledge—about anything, much less about health issues. We are in the middle of the greatest explosion of knowledge the world has ever seen. Information can go around the world with the speed of light. Go to the Internet and put in any health-related issue you can think of and up will come hundreds of sites where you can get information. Of course, you have to be careful what kind of information you are accessing and using, because anyone can post anything he or she likes on the Internet and some of what shows up there is useless and even dangerous information. Once again, rely on the Holy Spirit to guide you to the best sources of information.

Bookstores have huge sections crammed with health-related and weight-loss information, or go to the public library for a lot of free health information.

There are at least a dozen health-related magazines that have current and updated information with every issue. The same cautions you use to access Internet sites apply to choosing books and magazines to read. Be careful what you put into your mind. Choose that which "renews" the mind.

What to Do with This Knowledge

What should you do with all the knowledge you've gained through reading this book and others? Start to put the information into practice. No more *mañana* (tomorrow) diets. No more Monday diets—you know the ones: KFC on Sunday complete with chicken skin, mashed potatoes and gravy with the justification, "Tomorrow morning, baby, no more mashed potatoes and gravy for me. I'll kick it into high gear once I get beyond this last fling."

Once I got serious, I knew I had to start my healthy eating on Sunday or whatever day comes before *mañana*. No more excuses. No more procrastination. James 4:17 says, "To him who knows to do good and does not do it, to him it is sin." So what you do with your newly acquired knowledge is to put it to work creating a better body for God. Stop making the wrong choices. Stop making excuses. Start today to become a better you.

If You Are Still Asking Why You Need to Change

You will have to recognize that this is going to be a fight. You will get hungry. You will get lazy. You will want to give up. That's the time to remind yourself why you are doing this at all. Remember:

- You'll feel better.
- You'll have more energy.
- You'll have fewer pains.
- You'll look better.
- You'll gain strength spiritually.
- You'll live as if your body is the temple of God.

A Bod4God Close-Up

Mike Vencion
Lost 103 pounds

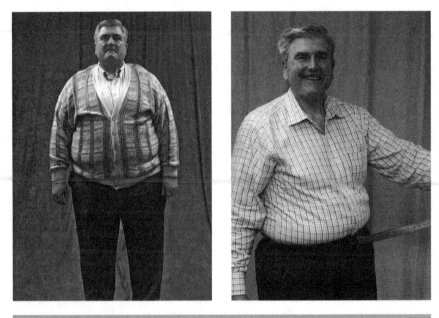

Before   **After**

My weight-loss miracle was a card that came from Pastor Steve advertising Bod4God. My father got the card and signed me up. I had played
semi-pro football and had earned a red belt in Karate. Then I gained so
much weight I could hardly move. Once, I wanted to see *The Lion King*
at Kennedy Center with my grandson, but I didn't go, because I
couldn't fit into the seat. Maybe I didn't realize how bad my situation
was, but my father did, and that's why he signed me up.

When I first walked through the door of the church, I felt awkward.
I had been raised in the Lutheran church and only came to this Baptist
Church because of the weight-loss competition. The first week I was

devastated when I weighed in. When you come in at more than 300 pounds and only lose two pounds, it seems you will never achieve all the weight loss needed. Then, all of a sudden, one Sunday I realized my whole life had changed. It was biblical principles that were making weight loss possible for me and those principles were affecting every part of my life. It became more than about losing weight.

My wife and I exercise every night. We both go to the gym. It has brought us closer together. Of course, it hasn't all been easy. There are setbacks and I haven't stopped loving to eat. I fight emotional eating. I'm in the insurance industry and it has been seriously affected by the economy. It is a temptation to overeat to ease the pain of the struggle. One thing I have done that helps is to keep a journal. I write down where I've been in my journey. I don't want to gain that weight back. The journal keeps me on focus.

I was drinking six to eight sugared soft drinks a day. I stopped drinking them cold turkey and started drinking water. Now I crave water. I started eating breakfast in the morning. I eat oatmeal and other whole-grain cereals. I started feeling better right away. I also started exercising. I started parking at the far end of the parking lot, and I started using the stairs. I use an elliptical machine for walking, and I use the time on the machine to pray.

The team competitions have meant a lot to me. They have taught me humility. The team meeting is the place where I get emotional stability to lose weight. The people here are unique and diverse.

Since I've lost weight, I've earned a wonderful reward. My grandson said, "For the first time I can put my arms around you." My inspiration for losing weight was to be here for my grandchildren. I don't ever want to gain back the weight I've lost. Some people carry before and after pictures. I keep my belt and wear it. I have more holes punched as I drop weight. It has turned into a sort of wraparound belt. It's a very visual way for me to keep track of my weight loss and remind me never to go back to where I once was.

Small Steps to Life Ideas

What Do You Need to Know About H$_2$O?

Additional considerations for drinking an adequate amount of water include the following:

- Water assists in absorption, digestion and metabolism of food because our bodies' proteins and enzymes work more efficiently in diluted solutions
- Drinking lots of water results in more muscle mass because our muscles are composed primarily of water
- Water gives you the energy and hydration needed for exercise
- When adequate amounts of water are not consumed, our bodies hold on to excess water for survival, causing bloating

Small Food Steps

Eat with people who have small appetites and observe how they eat. They probably put their fork down between bites. They probably only have one small serving of the foods they eat. They may turn down dessert, but if they are served dessert, they will probably only take a couple of bites. After all, the first bite tastes the best. At the same time, don't eat with people who encourage you to overeat. Probably some of those people are overweight. Fat friends support each others' bad eating habits. They too are toxic to you.

Small Exercise Steps

Remember that muscle burns calories even when the body is at rest. It's something like the idling engine of a car. It doesn't burn as much fuel in neutral, sitting in the driveway, as it does running at 70 miles per hour down the highway. Your muscle won't burn as much fat when you are resting, but it burns something. That's better than nothing. Get that muscle growing.

Small Steps to Life Record

What "Skinny Things" Will You Do this Week?

Fill out this chart each week by indicating: (1) What you will do to eat less to live; (2) What you will do to exercise more to live; and (3) What average daily ounces of water you will drink. Pick only a few things, and stick with them. Remember that weight loss and maintenance requires you to *eat less* and *exercise more*.

Sun.	
Mon.	
Tues.	
Wed.	
Thurs.	
Fri.	
Sat.	

Bod4God Victory Guide

To apply the information in this chapter to your life, work through the Victory Guide. It will equip you to practice the four keys to weight loss. Big losers make the Victory Guide a high priority. Record this week's weight change on "My Progress Report" located in appendix A.

Week Six: *I* Is for More Inspiration

Memory Verse
"I can do all things through Christ who strengthens me" (Phil. 4:13).

Reflection/Application Questions

1. Paul believed he could do all things through the strength of Jesus Christ. Do you really believe that Christ will give you the strength to maintain a Bod4God lifestyle? Why or why not?

    YES because HE said so.

2. How will you apply this to your life this week? Read the passages in the following table and summarize each in your own words. Then go back and put a checkmark next to verses you find inspirational.

John 10:10	*Satan comes to destroy you*
Philippians 4:13	*Christ can do all things*
Colossians 1:16	*He creates good things*
Psalm 139:14	*Give thanks for your body*
Matthew 16:24-25	*Give up the junk*
James 4:17	*Do the right thing*
Galatians 5:16	*Meditate on the Spirit*
1 Corinthians 6:19-20	*Your body belongs to Christ!*

3. Proverbs 23:7 says, "As he thinks in his heart, so is he." Are you experiencing a balance between rejecting and perfecting your body? Explain your answer.

Yes, but not in all Areas

4. Why do you think the motivation to live a healthy lifestyle is often so difficult?

It goes against the flesh And socceital norm's.

5. What is your motivation for losing weight? To live longer? To look better? To feel better? Or something else? Explain your answer.

My Bod4God Journal

Teach me, O Lord, the way of Your statutes, and I shall keep it to the end.
PSALM 119:33

Record what God is telling you to do this week to apply the four keys to a better body.

Dedication: Honoring God with My Body

_____
_____
_____
_____
_____

Inspiration: Motivating Myself for Change

_____
_____
_____
_____
_____

Eat and Exercise: Managing My Habits

_____
_____
_____
_____

Team: Building My Circle of Support

_____
_____
_____
_____
_____

E Is for Eat

Each of you should know how to possess his own vessel in
sanctification and honor.
1 THESSALONIANS 4:4

You've probably heard the adage that if you fail to plan, you plan to fail. You can have all the goals in the world, but if you don't have a plan to reach them, you'll never reach your goals. In this chapter, I want to help you discover and create a feasible plan to achieve whatever goal God has placed on your heart.

Maybe you don't know what your goal should be. James 1:5 says, "If any of you lacks wisdom, let him ask of God, who gives to all liberally and without reproach, and it will be given to him." Whenever we are in a quandary, we can ask God for wisdom. I challenge you to do so as you create a plan to achieve your goal. Ask God to lead you. There are many plans to weight loss, sticking to a plan is the key to weight loss.

Choose a Plan That Is Best for You

One of the main reasons most people fail on traditional diet plans is that they are told to eat what other people choose for them to eat. This approach simply doesn't work for most people because we don't all have the same appetites, background or circumstances. Bod4God is about crafting your own plan that you will do gladly for the rest of your life.

Get a Multitude of Counsel

Start talking to people about all the options for weight loss so you can figure out what will work best for you. Listen to what worked for them. Read the weight-loss stories in this book. Consider how to adapt the program those successful losers used to your specific concerns and needs. Get input from lots of sources on your plan. This is a biblical concept as well. Proverbs 15:22 says, "Without counsel, plans go awry, but in the multitude of counselors they are established."

Don't Wait to Make Your Plan: Do It Now

Advance decision-making is critical to a healthy lifestyle. Yet another Proverb has really helped me here. "A prudent man foresees evil and hides himself, but the simple pass on and are punished" (Prov. 22:3). Healthy living requires foresight.

My life is busy, and I have to set a plan. If I don't plan ahead, any goal I have set for myself doesn't happen. Not too long ago, I went to a pastor's conference. I knew it would be held at a nice, fancy hotel where there would be a lot of food. I can't say I was perfect in sticking to my healthy living lifestyle, but I did pretty well. I knew I was going to be breaking my routine. I had to think, *You're going to have less control over food choices. Think about how you're going to deal with those potatoes when they're put in front of you. What are you going to do with them?* I exchanged them for salads. I usually decide what to order at a restaurant before going in. This really helps me to deal with a tempting menu.

Follow a Routine

When you start making changes, your body will probably resist change at first. If you get on a routine, your body will get used to it. Make healthy eating a major part of your routine. Eat smaller portions and let your body get used to less food.

Think about the law of sowing and reaping in relationship to your health. Galatians 6:8 says, "He who sows to his flesh will of the flesh reap corruption." If you sow to your flesh by eating anything you want to eat, and if you don't exercise, you're going to corrupt your body. But if you sow to the Spirit, you will reap life. Galatians 6:9 encourages us by saying, "Let us not grow weary while doing good, for in due season we shall reap if we do not lose heart."

It is important to encourage yourself, because when you begin to make changes, it is very hard to follow through. Those first few weeks and days are difficult. Be encouraged that repetition will train your body to perform new habits and crave new things. If you will hang in there, you can retrain your body.

I love what Paul said in 1 Corinthians 9:27, "I discipline my body and bring it into subjection." I have to train my body, and the good news is that when I do, a lot of the things I used to crave I no longer want. For example, when I woke up this morning, the first thing I craved was an apple and a glass of water. It hasn't always been that way. But now, around lunchtime, I crave a salad because most days I eat a grilled chicken salad for lunch. When I began my Bod4God quest, it was about meat and potatoes and, of course, ice cream. It was about as little exercise as possible. Now, I've found a plan and a path that works for me, and I'll never go back to the lifestyle I once had.

Making a lifestyle change with regard to what you will eat, demands some thought and study. The very foundation of building a healthy lifestyle is to realize that God gave you life and a body, and you're to take your life and body and please Him in the things you do with them. Since there are so many mentions of the body in the Bible, we can know for sure that God didn't leave us on this earth without direction as to how we should manage our body. Matthew 16:24-25 states it plainly: To gain our life, we have to lose it. I had to become a loser, and that's where the Losing to Live idea came from. We can't take the easy way out. We have to eat less and exercise more—it's that simple.

We know what we should do to have better health. It's self that gets in the way of doing it. Self wants to eat the foods that are not healthy. Self doesn't want to exercise. Self doesn't want to die daily. But it's the only way we can lose to live.

Obey the Bible

The secret to weight loss is that there is no secret. You simply have to eat less and exercise more. You have to face this reality and quit looking for a pill or potion to solve your weight loss need. So let's talk about the issue of managing your habits. Again the Bible comes to the rescue. The main verse that has helped me here is 1 Thessalonians 4:4. "Each of you should know how to possess his own vessel in sanctification and honor." In the beginning, I didn't know how to "possess" my own body—I didn't know how to manage it. I had to learn. We can all do better about the way we eat. We can all improve. But how? How do we make choices that are healthy? How do we learn what is best for us?

Proverbs 4:20-22 is helpful: "My son, give attention to my words, incline your ear to my sayings. Do not let them depart from your eyes; keep them in the midst of your heart; for they are life to those who find them, and health to all their flesh." The place to start with lifestyle changes is the Bible—the Word of God. There are two basic things that the Word of God teaches with regard to losing weight and having a healthy lifestyle. Here they are:

1. Eat in Moderation (see Proverbs 23:2)

For me, and for many of us who are overweight, that means eating less. For all of us it means making healthier eating choices. For someone who is anorexic, it will mean eating sensibly—the right things in the right portions to keep the body healthy.

2. Get the Right Amount of Exercise (see Genesis 2:15)

Overweight people don't want to hear that. We blame a low metabolism as the reason we can't lose weight, and it is probably true for many of us. But some of you are skinny and you have terrible eating habits. You are sneaking by because you have a high metabolism. While many overweight people envy you, you too may be a glutton. (Tough talk, huh.) I'm not a scientist or a nutritionist, but I know we can't use slow metabolism as an excuse to be overweight. We have to get our body moving. We have to exercise to get our metabolism going. If you do enough exercise and eat less, you will very likely lose weight.

How Then Shall You Eat?

The answer to what shall we eat is simple: *better* and *less*. Eat less and eat foods that are as close to the way God made them as possible—straight from the ground, straight from the trees. Eat food for health and not because you think it will make you happy.

God is one cool God. He created food and He wants us to enjoy our food. He put 10,000 taste buds on the tongue, in the throat and esophagus that provide information about the taste of the food we eat. Taste buds detect the four elements of taste perception: salty, sour, bitter, sweet. The food we eat hits clusters of these taste receptors and transfers the information to the cortex of the cerebrum in our brain. It's a complicated process that was given to us for one reason. God wants us to enjoy the taste of our food.

Food is beautiful—especially food in its natural state before all identity has been processed out of it. I suppose God could have made all our food gray in color and it could have been just as nutritious as it is now, but He didn't do that. He made orange food—carrots, pumpkins and citrus fruits. He made dark green leafy vegetables, some with red stems to appeal first to the eye and then to the palate. He made foods that are red and purple and white and yellow, and they are beautiful, and we want to eat them. Go to a food store that specializes in fresh fruits and vegetables—a place like Pike Place Market in Seattle, Washington, where fruits and vegetables are stacked on farmers tables like works of art, or a Whole Foods store found in many major cities where there are lovely piles of fresh food. Or visit a farmer's market or roadside stand in season and just enjoy the look of the beautiful food God has given us in its natural state. God wanted us to enjoy the way our food looks.

The Bible said of the children of Israel, "For the LORD your God is bringing you into a good land, a land of brooks of water, of fountains and springs, that flow out of valleys and hills; a land of wheat and barley, of vines and fig trees and pomegranates, a land of olive oil and honey" (Deut. 8:7-8). This was the Promised Land, and it was described by what they would get to eat once they got there. God was saying, "Get ready! The food is going to be great, and you're going to love it. There's going to be lots of clean, fresh water. It's going to spring up from deep springs. It's going to flow down from the mountains. Make your kitchen into the Promised Land!"

"But I don't do vegetables, and very little fruit, either," I hear you say. Well, that has to change. Remember that taste is acquired. There are places in the world where people eat grasshoppers and insect larvae.

There are places where people eat animals we consider pets. *And they enjoy what they eat!* Taste is something we learn from our parents and our culture. Some of our learning has not been particularly good for our health. We have to unlearn the kinds of eating behavior that hurt us and relearn healthier ways of eating. You can learn to eat fruits and vegetables and enjoy them—and you must.

Okay, let's get into it and talk about what kinds of foods to eat. While this program doesn't try to tell you what you can eat and what you can't eat, there are some guidelines that will help you. First and foremost, shop for "live" foods. Live foods are those found around the outside aisles of the grocery store. That's where you find the fruits, vegetables, dairy, meats, poultry and fish that are so healthy for us. Down the inside aisles is where you find processed foods that are certainly not alive, and perhaps they have been on those shelves for months or years. Do you really want to focus on putting that kind of food—food often loaded with preservatives—into your body?

We can't say a lack of information is responsible for the overweight condition in which we, as a nation, find ourselves. The U.S. Department of Agriculture (USDA) created an icon that serves as a reminder to help Americans make healthier food choices. The icon is shaped like a dinner plate in order to prompt people to think about building a healthy plate at mealtimes. At the USDA website www.ChooseMyPlate.gov, you will see the icon (pictured below), which illustrates the five food groups using a place

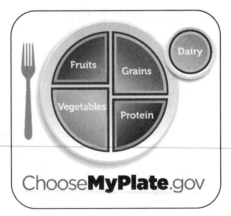

Image courtesy of the U.S. Department of Agriculture.
The USDA does not endorse any products, goods or services.

setting. At the website you can also find more information and tips about making healthy food choices.

Registered dietitian Emily Ann Miller states, "One thing that MyPlate reminds you to do is to make half of your plate fruits and vegetables. Almost any kind of fruit (fresh, frozen, canned, dried, or 100 percent fruit juice) is a good choice. A small amount of 100-percent fruit juice is okay and does provide some nutrients, but it does not provide the fiber that is necessary for good health the way that whole fruit does. Try to eat fruit in its whole state instead of drinking juice. When choosing canned fruit, look for fruits packed in 100 percent fruit juice or water instead of syrup, which has a lot of added sugar. Vegetables may be raw or cooked; fresh, frozen, canned, or dried/dehydrated. Choose a variety of colorful veggies; the USDA website has many ideas for including vegetables into your meals every day.

"MyPlate shows that you should fill approximately one-quarter of your plate with grains. Any food made from wheat, rice, oats, cornmeal, barley or another cereal grain is a grain product. Examples include bread, pasta, oatmeal, breakfast ceareals, tortillas and grits. Aim to choose whole grains for at least half of the grains you eat each day. Whole grains are made with the entire grain kernel and are more nutritious than refined grains such as white bread or white rice.

"Proteins, which should take up approximately one-quarter of your plate, include meat, poultry, seafood, beans and peas, eggs, processed soy products, nuts, and seeds. Meat and poultry choices should be lean or low fat. Look for leaner cuts of meat, such as sirloin or round steak. If meats are marbled with fat, they are not lean. Always trim off all visible fat. Seafood and plant proteins (soy, nuts, seeds, beans, and peas) are good protein alternatives to meat and poultry choices. Always bake, broil or grill meat, poultry, and seafood instead of frying it, which adds a lot of calories and unhealthy fat.

"Finally, the MyPlate icon includes the dairy group. All fluid milk products and many foods made from milk are considered part of this food group. Look for fat-free or low-fat dairy food choices, such as 1 percent or skim milk. Whole milk is not recommended for adults and children past the age of two years because of the unhealthy fat content. Dairy products are a great source of calcium, so if you don't drink milk or eat dairy products, you will need to look for other foods with high calcium content."

The www.ChooseMyPlate.gov website has many tools for learning how to eat in a healthy manner. It's free, so use it to your health's advantage. Most of the information found there works well when you are at home. It's not too hard to keep track of what you are putting in your mouth when you are at home. Where you get into trouble is when you eat out. It used to be that Americans rarely ate out, but now most Americans eat out three or four times a week.

Learn to Read Labels

Learn to read nutrition labels on the back of food packages. You won't find nutrition labels on things like apples, apricots and avocados, but they are on anything humans have processed. The government requires the food label to be there.

Calories per Serving

The first thing to look at when reading a label is the portion size. Many people don't consider this and think they are taking in fewer calories than they really are because instead of eating a half-cup serving of something, they have eaten a cup.

Then check out the calories in a single serving. Calories are fuel for the body and we need them to live, but if we have become overweight, it's an indication we have consistently taken in more calories than we can burn and the excess is being stored as fat. If you're going to lose weight, you are going to have to cut back on calories.

Fats

Next look at the fat grams. Fat is dense, and a little fat can pack a lot of calories. There are healthy fats and there are dangerous trans fats. Trans fat is the common name for a type of unsaturated fat with *trans*-isomer fatty acid. These fats can increase the risk of heart disease by raising LDL (bad cholesterol) and lowering HDL (good cholesterol).

There are some who have tried to eliminate all fats from their diet. It's not a smart thing to do. Everyone needs some fat in their diet to maintain healthy cells, a strong nervous system and good skin and hair. However, these fats should be mono-unsaturated fats such as those found in nuts, olive oil and other unsaturated oils. Omega 3 oils, found in fish, nuts and olive oil, for example, are necessary for good health.

The healthy kind of fats are necessary for the ultimate functioning of the body and mind. They promote a healthy heart. They help prevent cancer. They keep down inflammation. They benefit nerve cells in the eyes and promote eye health. Because the brain is 60 percent fat, fat is necessary for healthy communication between the brain and nervous system. The right fats improve your mood and help in weight loss by increasing satisfaction from the foods you eat so that you will eat less. Unfortunately, the body does not differentiate between types of fats, and so all fats—good and bad—contribute to weight. We need healthy oils, but we need them in moderation.

Fiber

Check out the fiber grams on the label. You want to choose foods with a high fiber content, as most Americans don't eat enough fiber. You need 30 grams of fiber every day to keep the body functioning at its optimum. Here are some words of advice from Dr. Darren Baroni, board certified gastroenterologist:

> Eating fiber is very important to digestive tract health and general health overall. The more insoluble fiber that is in a person's diet, the less time bowel waste (and potential cancer causing substances called carcinogens) spend in the small intestine and colon. Fiber has been shown to be protective against colon cancer and probably against precancerous polyps. Additionally, fiber is more filling then other food ingredients and because, for the most part, it cannot be fully digested is lower in its overall caloric content. Hmmm, food that fills you up but is not high in calories—doesn't that sound like a perfect food? This is not surprising given it comes from a perfect Creator! Foods high in fiber are whole grains, raw fruits and most vegetables.
>
> Limit your intake not only of fat, but also of sodium and cholesterol. Pick those foods with high Vitamin A and C. They are good choices. Look also for calcium and iron contents.

Every food label also has a Daily Values column. While this is helpful information, remember that what you find there is a percentage of what you should have for the whole day and it is based on a 2,000 calorie a day diet.

Look at the ingredients list. Ingredients are listed in descending order by weight. If sugar is the first ingredient, it is the heaviest ingredient and you are buying little more than sugar in that product. Sugar may also be called "corn syrup," "dextrose," "glucose" or other words ending in "-ose."

Make wise choices with your food purchases. Truly read those labels and know what you are putting in your mouth. It matters. It makes a difference, and the difference shows up in added weight or loss of weight.[1]

How Much Shall You Eat?

You need to eat enough to fuel your body so that it is at peak efficiency for what God wants you to do in life. God intended that you glorify him with your body in your eating. First Corinthians 10:31 says, "Whether you eat or drink, or whatever you do, do all to the glory of God." Even your eating can glorify God. Maybe the last time you went to church you said, "I'm going to go worship and glorify God." That's wonderful! But in the same way, you can glorify Him when you go to lunch after church. I'll be honest: I'm not sure about all the ways you can glorify God by what you eat, but I am sure that overeating and gluttony are not among them (see Prov. 23:1-3).

Some time ago, I was asked, "What would Jesus eat?" I thought about that question and decided He was probably not a vegetarian (see John 21:12-13; Luke 15:23). I don't think He would overeat, either. I think He would have eaten the diet of the culture, but in moderation. And we already know He exercised, because He walked everywhere He needed to go.

Water, Water, Water

Many people, like Carol Thompson, don't drink a lot of water. Rather they drink sugar-loaded soft drinks. Carol is easily fatigued and she found that soft drinks with sugar made her feel better. It was addictive. She drank about four soft drinks a day to get a boost. She has since learned that not only do these sugared drinks cause one to be overweight, but they are also bad for your joints.

"I finally realized that all that sugar in the colas was affecting my weight. I stopped drinking them and looked for something to replace them." Carol said. "In the beginning, I drank fruit juices. Then I looked for something to drink that has protein. I began to drink Glucerna and other meal replacement drinks. The problem was that they too have lots of sugar. Then I began to drink a lot more water. It satisfies my cravings. Probably the biggest reason why I lost 15 pounds during my weight-loss competition was that I gave up drinking sugared colas."

Carol learned that water can be more satisfying than sugared soft drinks. Let's talk some more about water and its importance to life. Water is the most common and important liquid on Earth. Seventy percent of the earth's surface is covered with water. Life is impossible without it, and all known forms of life depend on it.

In the body, water works to transport nutrients and oxygen all through the body. It functions as a lubricant and a coolant. It is used for respiration, regulating the body's temperature, increasing metabolism and is necessary for the removal of body wastes.

In addition, water maintains muscle tone, gives us clear and healthy skin and, of course, assists in weight loss. It helps prevent lower back pain, chronic fatigue, headaches and migraines, asthma, allergies, arthritis, rheumatoid arthritis, hypertension, cholesterol, muscle pain, neck pain, joint pain, constipation, ulcers, stomach pain, confusion and disorientation, and there is even some research that ties lack of water intake to Alzheimers' Disease. More research with regard to the Alzheimers' connection is needed, but it is something to watch.

Water is a great aid in losing weight because it is calorie-free, has no fat or cholesterol and is low in sodium. Water acts as an appetite suppressant, decreases fat deposits, increases muscle mass, keeps the kidneys functioning properly and minimizes water retention.

Healthy kidneys can filter more than 500 ounces of water a day, but the highest recommended daily allowance in moderate climates is

129 ounces a day. Remember that only about 20 percent of your recommended daily allowance of water comes from other beverages and foods.

To help you increase your intake of water, start the day with a glass of water. Then throughout the day, don't wait until you are thirsty to drink. If you're thirsty, you are already dehydrated. Set a timer to drink water throughout the day. Add ice or lemon to your drink if you like. And choose vegetables every day that are high in water content.

What to Do When You Want to Cheat

The Bible tells us that the very first temptation ever was one involving food. Submitting to temptation with regard to food is as old as the Garden of Eden. "So when the woman saw that the tree was good for food, that it was pleasant to the eyes, and a tree desirable to make one wise, she took of its fruit and ate. She also gave to her husband with her, and he ate" (Gen. 3:6).

There it is. Eve looked, she saw, she desired it, she ate, she gave it to Adam. We haven't progressed very far from that scenario. We look, we see, we want it, we eat it and we may give it to someone else, causing him or her to give in to temptation as well. Eve's battle was to not eat the fruit. Our battle is to eat fruit. Many of us don't like fruit, but that's because we've not made eating fruit a habit.

If we are overweight, we have a huge challenge. Because we are creatures of habit, our bodies resist change. And when we finally do make a change, our bodies want to revert to the old ways. I know this is true. I had a habit of eating ice cream every night for 48 years. I probably didn't go to bed more than 10 times without eating ice cream. I had a deeply ingrained habit that was hard for me to break. Here's what I did.

When I started Bod4God, I had a cheat *meal*. Not a cheat day or week—a cheat meal on Friday night. Just one meal. When I had a craving—maybe on Tuesday—I postponed that craving to eat at my cheat meal on Friday night. I looked forward to that time when I could have the pizza I had been craving all week. The cheat meal was a big help to me in retraining my eating habits. I don't need a cheat meal now because I've changed. You may be trying hard to change, but you're not there yet, and so you need a cheat meal.

You have to bring your body into subjection. You can do this. Did you know that taste is developed? It is a learned behavior. You might not have a taste for healthy food, but you *can* change that. In Mark 1:6, we learn that John the Baptist ate locust and wild honey. How would you like a nice plate of locusts with honey drizzled all over it. It looks gross to me, but if John were here, he probably wouldn't want a quarter pounder with cheese, or Breyer's ice cream. He would prefer his locust and honey because that's what he learned to like.

It's time to tell your body what it's going to do rather than letting it tell you what it wants. You might not like water, but if you keep drinking your full quota of water every day, you will develop a taste for it. Claim the promises found in 1 Corinthians 10:13, which says, "No temptation has overtaken you except such as is common to man; but God is faithful, who will not allow you to be tempted beyond what you are able, but with the temptation will also make the way of escape, that you may be able to bear it." Will you choose to take the way of escape?

Three Things to Do When You Want to Cheat

1. Pray Consistently

You have to understand that part of overcoming temptation involves prayer. Luke 18:1 says, "Men always ought to pray, and not lose heart." Your choices are to pray and be victorious or not pray and faint. Pray about your exercise. Pray about your eating habits. Tell God that you've stopped looking for the quick fix—the magic pill—and you are ready to let Him help you. He will.

Be proactive and pray positively for healthy habits and not just negatively for your health problems. When I ask people what are their prayer needs, often what I hear in response is an "organ recital." You know, "I have a weak kidney," or, "I have diabetes," or, "The doctor is worried about my heart." It would be so exciting to hear, "Pastor, pray for me to drink more water." That would be a positive, preventive prayer of faith.

2. Shop Carefully

The rule of thumb is this: If food gets near you, it will eventually get in you. The battleground is not your kitchen—it's the grocery store. Shop for your health, not your happiness. If you keep what you shouldn't eat out of you basket, you'll keep it out of your car; and if you keep it out of the car, you'll keep it out of your house. I've literally stood at the check-out counter and thought, *What am I doing with this food?* I've sent it back rather than take it to the car and home. In Romans 13:14, Paul says, "Put on the Lord Jesus Christ, and make no provision for the flesh, to fulfill its lusts." Here are some tips for healthy grocery shopping:

- Don't go shopping when you are hungry. The temptation may just be too great.
- Pray for the filling of the Holy Spirit before you go into the store. I pray, "Oh God, fill me right now." I don't want to fulfill the lust of my flesh.
- Remember to shop on the outside aisles of the store where the living food is.
- Take the time to read the labels. Know what's in what you eat.
- Purchase some healthy snacks. I like fruit and almonds. Almonds are a plant-based protein high in fiber. They are filling and satisfying and help to promote good heart health. I eat a handful every day.

3. Think Correctly

In 2 Corinthians 10:4-5, Paul says, "The weapons of our warfare are not carnal, but mighty through God to the pulling of down strong holds; casting down imaginations, and every high thing that exalteth itself against the knowledge of God, bringing every into captivity every thought to the obedience of Christ" (*KJV*). In this case, and for us, "imaginations" are food cravings. What happens is that we start thinking about our cravings. If we don't cast down our imaginations—clear out our mind and let the Holy Spirit take control—we will give in to our cravings. Remember that every sin begins in the mind. We can't afford to let sinful thoughts stay in our mind.

There is a kind of detrimental thinking I call "Esau think." In Genesis 25 we find the story of Esau, who had been out hunting all day. He came to Jacob and said, "Please feed me with that same red stew, for I am weary." Jacob took advantage of the situation and replied, "Sell me your birthright." In that culture, the elder son took precedence over his younger brother. After the father's death, he would acquire a double portion of inheritance. Esau ignored all of that and said, "Look, I am about to die; so what is this birthright to me?" He sold it right then and there.

The Bible doesn't let it go. Hebrews 12:16 calls Esau a profane person who sold his birthright for one morsel of meat. Esau could have so much, but he gave it all up for a dish of soup. He thought he had to have short-term pleasure and it was worth more than his inheritance. What about your health? You know that some of the stuff you put in your mouth is not good for you. You know it and yet you do it.

Instead of "Esau" faith, we need to have "Moses" faith. Moses' parents feared God more than they feared Pharaoh. They hid him until they just couldn't hide him any longer. Later, when Moses came of age, he refused to live in Pharaoh's house. To Moses, short-term pleasure was not worth the long-term pain of seeing his people suffer. Don't be fooled. Sin is fun—for a season. Moses made the choice (see Heb. 11:24-27). He walked away from everything because he had right thinking. In the midst of plenty such as we have in this country, you have to remember that long-term health is not worth the short-term pleasure of junk food.

My friends, failure is not final. If you cheat—learn from it. Get back on track right away. The Bible says, "For a righteous man may fall seven times and rise again" (Prov. 24:16). Ninety percent of life is just showing up. You've showed up. You're here. Keep showing up. Keep taking those small steps to health.

Note
1. Dr. Baroni, personal correspondence to the author, Tuesday March 17, 2009. Used by permission.

Before   **After**

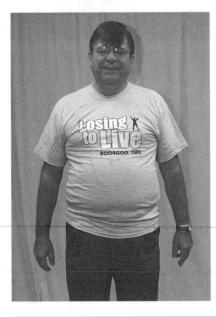 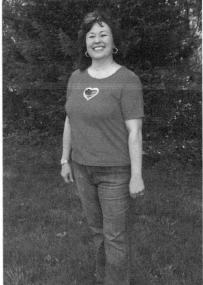

Before   **After**

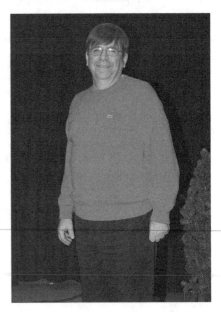

A Bod4God Close-Up

Gail Mates Pavlik
Lost 50 pounds

I have been overweight my whole life. Mom wanted me to stay slim. In the second grade she put me on a diet. I won many awards, some as a majorette. Mom also wanted me to be in a pageant, and when I wasn't the "ideal weight," she made me stay in until I was at the weight she wanted me to be. Mom's putting me on a diet only made me want to eat more. Food was my comfort. I worshiped food. I lived to eat. My eating was definitely emotional.

Of course, I soon became overweight. I had sleep apnea, high cholesterol and my good cholesterol was nonexistent. I had metabolic syndrome, pre-diabetes and high triglycerides. My father's poor health history was staring me in the face.

I went to Weight Watchers numerous times, had shots, took diet pills—the whole gamut of weight-loss possibilities. I was a fanatic about getting thin back then. Today, I just want to be healthy. Sometimes when I was overweight, I wanted to hide from everyone. When I came to this program, I wondered if it could be any different.

There was a time in my life when I taught two aerobics classes. I could motivate others but not myself. Then, Patricia Dutchie, my Losing to Live leader, made me commit to what she felt I could do. I began taking small steps to life. Sugar-loaded cherry soft drinks were my caffeine drug of choice. I had to stop drinking them.

It's not the big changes that I have made that are helping me lose weight, but rather the small steps. It's the power of God that has changed me. I have learned that the team approach is everything. The group leader and team members call and check on me to see how I'm doing. My team prays with me and I pray with my team for God to give us strength to stick to the plan all week. It works for me.

My life has been dramatically changed through Bod4God. These small steps to life have since led to me being chosen as a Go Red For Women national spokeswoman with the American Heart Association.

Tom Pavlik
Lost 22 pounds

I weighed 132 lbs. when I graduated from college. I weighed 247 when I started Bod4God. In the past my weight-controlling exercise had always been running six miles a day on the treadmill. Then I blew out my knee and had to have surgery. The doctors said I should not do any more distance running, so I stopped *all* exercise—and I gained weight.

When I married Gail, we ate out a lot. We enjoyed food and we gained weight. We tried many times to lose weight and between us have lost hundreds of pounds together, but we've gained them all back. We were in that lose/gain cycle for four years. Every time I gained, I gained more weight than I had lost when dieting. I struggled psychologically, telling myself that I was just getting old. I wasn't motivated to get my weight down.

Then came Bod4God. This program works because you don't have to sacrifice. We didn't have to cheat a part of ourselves. I have never felt that I was denying myself on this program. Gail and I just got into a better balance. I hate counting points or calories, and in this program you don't have to count. We began making small changes rather than huge ones, and that worked. The body resists change, so it will resist any major change, but it will accept small changes.

After the surgery, the doctor said that my knee worked fine and I needed to go back to the gym. I began to focus again on exercise. I was afraid, though, that the knee wouldn't work. It was tough to get started. My knee would swell and I'd ice it down after exercise. Now, since I've lost weight, my knee is much better. I'm trying to do an hour a day on the treadmill, five days a week.

Because of my job, I have to eat out. When I'm out, I now eat fish since it is healthier and has less calories. I love bread. There was a time when I could eat a loaf of bread at a sitting. I try to replace bread and potatoes with veggies. Now Gail and I split appetizers and meals. Gail thought I was trying to save money or hold out on her or something by doing this. But I wasn't. We simply had to eat less, and it has worked for both of us.

Small Steps to Life Ideas

Have you weighed in? How are you doing? If you have been faithful to the Small Steps to Life, you have probably lost some weight—maybe even a lot of weight.

What Do You Need to Know About H$_2$O?

This chapter has a lot more good information about water. Don't neglect to drink an adequate amount of water every day. Let's stop and thank God for water. "Thank You, God, for rain and ice and snow. Bless you, Father, for being Jehovah Jirah, the God who provides water so we can drink what we need and take care of our bodies. Amen."

Small Food Steps

Plan your snacks. Successful dieters eat about six small meals a day to maintain their metabolism. Eating small meals like this keeps a steady flow of glucose to the body. Here are some ideas for eating more healthy snacks:

- Spread a tablespoon of peanut butter on apple slices.
- Toss dried cranberries and chopped nuts—walnut or almond—in a bowl of instant oatmeal.
- Top fat-free or lowfat vanilla yogurt with crunchy granola—a tablespoon or two—and add blueberries.
- Have fat-reduced microwave popcorn and sprinkle it with a bit of Parmesan cheese for flavor, but do not add butter or margarine.
- Put nonfat frozen whipped topping between two graham or chocolate graham crackers for an "ice-cream sandwich."
- Dip bits and pieces of veggies in nonfat dressing.
- Dip strawberries or apple slices in nonfat yogurt.

Small Exercise Steps

Learn some exercises you can do at your desk or while traveling in a car or airplane. Do some leg lifts by lifting your feet off the ground and hold them up for a few seconds while tightening your abs. Do this several times a day for several weeks and you will begin to have tighter abs. Remember that muscle burns fat even when your body is at rest.

Small Steps to Life Record

What "Skinny Things" Will You Do this Week?

Fill out this chart each week by indicating: (1) What you will do to eat less to live; (2) What you will do to exercise more to live; and (3) What average daily ounces of water you will drink. Pick only a few things, and stick with them. Remember that weight loss and maintenance requires you to *eat less* and *exercise more*.

Sun.	
Mon.	
Tues.	
Wed.	
Thurs.	
Fri.	
Sat.	

Bod4God Victory Guide

To apply the information in this chapter to your life, work through the Victory Guide. It will equip you to practice the four keys to weight loss. Big losers make the Victory Guide a high priority. Record this week's weight change on "My Progress Report" located in appendix A.

Week Seven: *E* Is for Eat

Memory Verse

"Each of you should know how to possess his own vessel in sanctification and honor" (1 Thess. 4:4).

Reflection/Application Questions

1. What does Paul mean in 1 Thessalonians 4:4 when he writes, "Each of you should know how to possess his own vessel"?

   _____

   _____

   _____

   _____

   _____

   _____

   _____

   _____

2. What is the connection between obedience to God and managing your eating habits?

   _____

   _____

   _____

   _____

   _____

   _____

   _____

   _____

3. We often find ways to abuse God's perfect gifts, such as food. In what ways have you abused God's gift of food?

    _____

    _____

    _____

    _____

    _____

    _____

    _____

    _____

4. In what ways are you using food to meet needs other than nourishment in your life?

    _____

    _____

    _____

    _____

    _____

    _____

    _____

5. Gluttony is an action that reflects a person who is controlled by appetite. When are you most vulnerable to gluttony?

    _____

    _____

    _____

    _____

    _____

    _____

    _____

6. What foods tempt you the most?

_____
_____
_____
_____
_____
_____
_____
_____
_____
_____

7. What steps do you need to take to make sure you are consuming enough water each day?

_____
_____
_____
_____
_____
_____
_____
_____
_____
_____

My Bod4God Journal

Teach me, O Lord, the way of Your statutes, and I shall keep it to the end.
PSALM 119:33

Record what God is telling you to do this week to apply the four keys to a better body.

Dedication: Honoring God with My Body

_____
_____
_____
_____
_____

Inspiration: Motivating Myself for Change

_____
_____
_____
_____
_____

Eat and Exercise: Managing My Habits

_____
_____
_____
_____

Team: Building My Circle of Support

_____
_____
_____
_____
_____

E Is for Exercise

Therefore, whether you eat or drink, or whatever you do,
do all to the glory of God.
1 CORINTHIANS 10:31

Do I have to exercise for the rest of my life? Yes, you do. There is no way around the fact that permanent weight loss only comes to those who exercise. Eighty-five-year-old Bob McAllister of our congregation is one of the most active guys in the whole Bod4God program. He goes to the gym three days a week, works out on the equipment for a half-hour before going to aerobics class, then cycles and does other exercises as well. The exercise, combined with eating smaller portions, helped him lose 26 pounds in 20 weeks.

Read any of the stories in this book and you will soon see that eating less and exercising more are the keys to health and a trim body.

Exercise in Bod4God simply means moving your body. That doesn't mean you have to join a body builders class or spend all day at the gym exercising. There are Small Steps to Life you can do that begin to benefit your body right away. What's encouraging is that all of the people in our stories began to feel better when they shed a few pounds and got moving.

Pete Frenquelle, whose story is told at the end of this chapter, said a mouthful when he said: "As far as exercise, what I've learned is that the more you gain, the more you hate to move. The more you hate to move, the more you gain. The more weight you lose, the more you want to move. The more you feel like moving, the more you lose." It's so simple, but so true.

When Did Exercise Become a Problem?

God made man to be physically active. When God created man, as recorded in Genesis 2, He put him in a garden and said, "Get to work. Tend the garden." If you've ever done extensive gardening, you know that it exercises every muscle in your body. I'm sure that there were vines to be cut back, crops to be harvested and perhaps even seeds to be planted.

Then, when Adam and Eve sinned and were driven from the Garden of Eden, their work *truly* began. Now they had to fight the earth. God said, "In the sweat of your face you shall eat bread" (Gen. 3:19). Things were not going to come easily to this couple anymore, and things don't come easily to us either. We have to work for what we get.

God intended us to be physically active. In the last 100 years, things have changed. We have gone from being an industrial society to being a technological society. We've gone from 15-hour days in the field to 15-hour days in front of a computer screen. We've gone from being physically active to being physically inactive. And it hasn't done our society any good. The sedentary lifestyle most of us now follow has contributed to the problem of obesity in this country. It's shocking to read that a Johns Hopkins study predicts that by the year 2048, every American adult could be overweight; and within 21 years, one out of every six health-care dollars spent will be attributable to obesity.

There is nothing wrong with doing sedentary work as long as you realize you have to compensate for the lack of exercise in your line of work by being intentional about exercise. You have to schedule exercise into your life or it won't happen. I'm sure there are heads nodding everywhere. You know what I mean, don't you?

There is only one Scripture in the Bible that mentions the word "exercise." It is found in 1 Timothy 4:8, where Paul writes to Timothy, "For bodily exercise profits a little." I loved this verse, and if anybody talked about exercise, I would remind those people that it only profited "a little." However, that verse is a comparative statement. It is comparing physical exercise with spiritual exercise. When we exercise physically, we are taking care of the temporal. When we exercise spiritually, we're taking care of the eternal.

Some of you are out of balance in this area. Some of you are physically active and in perfect shape, but you never read your Bible, pray, or go to church as you should. You have abs and biceps to prove that you are strong physically, but you don't have the spiritual muscles you need to survive in this world. You need to exercise spiritually. All of us will die one day, and we'd better be investing ourselves in something that's going to outlast us, something of eternal significance. That's what the Timothy verse is teaching us. We can't use that verse as an excuse not to exercise, because God has told us to be physically active. We have to become more intentional about getting enough exercise.

By the way, look again at that verse in 1 Timothy. Paul doesn't say that exercise profits us nothing. He says it does profit us, but only a little compared to the pursuit of spiritual strength. We need both physical exercise and spiritual exercise. The Olympic Games began hundreds of years before the time that Paul wrote those words in his letter to Timothy. The Romans and the Greeks were seriously into games where physical strength and endurance was essential, and lack of strength and endurance often cost players their lives. But what was the *spiritual* strength of these athletes? In many cases, it was probably nonexistent. The players were probably worshipers of both the gods and the emperor.

So if you are one of those people who have a great physique, but you never look between the covers of your Bible, and you never pray, remember that bodily exercise only profits "a little."

What Are the Benefits of Exercise?

The benefits of exercise are multiple. Exercise helps your body in almost every conceivable way. One of the greatest benefits of exercise is that it helps you lose weight. Only a small percentage of people can lose weight without exercise; but 100 percent of people have to exercise to be healthy. Remember that in the time of the Bible, people had no cars. They walked with seemingly little regard for distance. While not having transportation may seem like a problem, for these people it was a blessing in disguise. They didn't have to go to the gym every day. They got plenty of exercise. On the other hand, we don't walk everywhere like that and we have to make sure that we are exercising enough to gain benefits from it.

The most important step in establishing a fitness program is to do *something*. You can choose any kind of exercise that works for you. You can do cardio/strength or strength and flexibility programs. You can decide if you want to work with a group or do it alone. Many people exercise alone, but there is nothing like working out and exercising with a buddy to keep you on task and accountable.

Ask yourself the question, "What sabotages my attempts to exercise?" Make whatever that thing is a matter of prayer and planning.

You need to start exercising slowly. If you go all out on your first day and then become so sore you can't exercise again the next day, you haven't gained much. Remember, this is a lifestyle change, and real change can come slowly. Make sure you stretch before exercising to prevent injury and prevent soreness. Keep track of how often you exercise. Keep your exercise routine simple. It might help to play music, perhaps praise songs, while you exercise. Maybe you can listen to a book on CD or iPod, or do your Scripture memory work while you are exercising. Vary your workout to use all seven muscle groups. This is called cross-training.

Exercise must become a habit—a sacred appointment you keep with yourself. God designed us to handle physical work. We were not fashioned to live sedentary lives filled with stress. So choose an active lifestyle.

How Much Exercise Is Enough?

If you have to ask that question, you are probably not getting enough exercise. One doctor recommends a 5/30 program (30 minutes 5 times each week). Other programs advocate exercise every day. For more information, check with your doctor or another health care provider.

Exercise books are a dime a dozen in secondhand shops, and they all say pretty much the same thing. So if you are strapped for cash, use your money to get a good pair of cross trainer shoes and pick up a secondhand book on exercise. You don't need a fancy gym membership, although many people enjoy the camaraderie they find in exercising with other folks. An exercise pal is a good thing to have; you can encourage each other to get going on days when one or the other doesn't feel like moving.

Our church partners with a ministry called Body & Soul, Where Faith and Fitness Meet (www.bodyandsoul.org) to offer an awesome exercise program that provides cardio and strength training fitness set to contemporary Christian music. Body & Soul was developed by fitness specialists Jeannie and Roy Blocher, in Germantown, Maryland.

This ministry equips fitness-minded Christians to lead exercise classes both in the church and in the community. They also provide an encouraging environment for Christians to improve their health and invite their non-Christian friends to do the same. Jeannie Blocher says, "Develop an exercise program that motivates you to do it day after day. You want to wake up each day saying about your exercise program, 'I can do that again today.' The most important thing about exercise is not what you do, but that you do it." Here are some of Jeannie's ideas:

- If you love the outdoors, walk, jog, bike, hike or Rollerblade™.
- If you want to pamper your joints and like the water, swim.
- Use a rocking chair instead of a regular chair.
- Find something you like to do that involves repetitious movement.
- Breathe deeply and forcefully several times a day to aerate your entire lungs.
- Go dancing, particularly square dancing, for fun and good exercise for all ages.
- Try a group fitness class, especially a faith-based one where you can find a safe, caring environment, whether you are a beginner or veteran exerciser.
- If you like competition, go for team sports—basketball, soccer or local softball teams.
- Have a family powwow where you decide how each member is going to participate in fitness.

- Plant the value of fitness in your kids at an early age and it will always be part of their lifestyle.
- Plan active vacations where you build some time away around physical activity.

The One Exercise That Fits All

Perhaps one of the easiest and best ways to get the exercise you need is to walk. The old Nike ad said it so clearly—"Just do it!" Just put on your shoes and get walking. Walking has so many benefits along with exercise. If you are having a relationship problem with someone, take a walk with him or her. It's a great opportunity to begin communication. Walking is a great time to pray. It's a great time to get out and enjoy nature.

Walking Clubs

Jesus walked with His disciples. Why not join a walking club and enjoy short walks and long hikes? A walking club will provide safety for members and encouragement from other walkers to keep exercising.

Our church has a walking club we call the "100-Mile Club." The goal is for participants to walk at least 100 miles over a 12-week period. We meet every Sunday evening for 12 weeks for a group walk. That gives a physical affirmation of our commitment to God, our bodies, our family and the Losing to Live fellowship.

We meet on the porch of the church to start our walk, and we walk the 5K route we will use for that event. We modify the course into A, B and C courses, depending on the walker's fitness level. The course is beautiful and God-inspired.

Mall Walking

Another walking option is mall walking. Many malls open their doors as early as 6:00 A.M. for people who want to use their facilities for exercise. People who walk in malls quickly get acquainted with each other and often form friendships. Usually, a regular walker will know how many laps of the mall you must take to walk a mile. You can walk early in the morning, any time during the day or in the early evening. But remember that there are peak times when the malls are crowded, and if you walk during those times, you will be constantly swerving to avoid shoppers. Mall walking provides shelter during rainy or wintry days, so there's no excuse to not walk!

Pedometers

If you are walking alone, a good way to motivate yourself is to buy a pedometer and use it every day. The goal should be 10,000 steps a day. It will take a while to build up to that number of steps, but it won't happen if you don't start.

Go to a high-end sporting goods store and invest in a good pedometer. Bad pedometers will only frustrate and discourage you as they do not accurately record your distance. (You can do online research for the various brands of pedometers available by typing the words "pedometer reviews" on a search engine.)

Shoes

Walking shoes are your most important item of gear, so plan to buy the best pair you can afford. You are worth the price. There is not a "best" shoe for everyone. The best shoe for you is the one that fits your foot and activity. If you've wondered whether to buy running shoes or walking shoes, buy the running shoes. That's because shoe manufacturers put their design resources into running shoes. Walking shoes are often little more than "pretty shoes."

If you start to take walking seriously and decide to walk in the mountains or go on a walking trip in this country or abroad, you might want to wear a boot. While boots are inflexible and heavy, they are great for walking on uneven surfaces such as you might find on a trail or on cobblestones in Europe. Boots protect the ankles from being turned and sprained.

Shop for shoes in the morning so that your feet will not be swollen. Take your time when buying walking shoes. Put on the shoes—both of them—and walk around the store for a while. Fitting problems should show up before you leave the store. When you get home, wear the shoes indoors for a few days in case you need to return them to the store.

Keep track of how many miles you have put on your shoes. They should be replaced before they have 600 miles on them because they lose their support. If you are overweight, are hard on your shoes or the shoes are lightweight, you may need to replace them closer to 300 miles. This is important, so even if your shoes don't look worn out, replace them anyway.

A good pair of walking shoes will probably cost $75 to $150. Remember, you are worth it and you can use the money you save by not buying a lot of expensive junk food.

What Are Some Other Ways to Exercise?

Do a few stretches early in the morning to get your metabolism started. Dance around while you brush your teeth. Do heel lifts while the coffee is brewing. Our Losing to Live participants find ways to exercise that better fit their unique lifestyles and schedules. Some people swim or work out at a gym facility. Sabrina Prime, a wife and mom who has lost 31 pounds, joined Bally's™ gym on a 90-day free offer coupon that was available when she signed up for the competition. She made such good use of the gym's offerings that she decided to rejoin when the 90 days were up.

Some participants get out and walk before breakfast. Some wait until just after breakfast. Some walk at noon when the day is the warmest. Some walk in the evening after work to get rid of tension. Some go to the gym. You have to find your own routine and stick to it.

Check off the small actions listed below that you can do right away to get started exercising and then make them part of your daily life just like brushing your teeth or combing your hair. The most important thing is that you take your exercise just as you would take a prescription:

- Do it three to five times a week—regularly.
- Pick a partner or exercise buddy to stay motivated.
- Plan ahead and set aside a regular exercise time.
- Keep track of your exercise program and be proud of yourself every day that you do it.

- Update your friends and family on your successes.
- Train, don't strain. Start slowly and gradually build up.
- Watch your diet and eat wisely.

A great website with video demonstrations of various exercises and other recommendations to get started *and* stay motivated is at the Centers of Disease Control (CDC): http://www.cdc.gov/physicalactivity/grow ingstronger/exercises/index.html.

Setting Exercise Goals

You need two kinds of goals: goals of output and goals of input. Let me explain. I set out to lose 100 pounds. That was my goal of output. But to reach that goal, I had to have a goal of input. I had to drink the water I was supposed to drink. I had to exercise at least three times a week. I had to eat properly. These were my goals of input. So, too, must you establish goals of input to achieve your output goal.

Additionally, it helps to recognize that your output goal is a statement of faith in God's ability to help you achieve it. When you state your goal, say it in faith. "I will lose 30 pounds by Thanksgiving." Jesus said about faith that we are to say to the mountain, "Be removed" (Matt. 21:21). You have to have faith that you will have a healthier future. You are painting a vision of what you want your life to look like.

In Habakkuk 2:2, God instructed the prophet, "Write the vision and make it plain on tablets, that he may run who reads it." Can I remind you again to write down your exercise goal and put it where you can see it? Keep your goal in front of you.

Now, let's talk for a moment about goal setting.

1. An exercise goal must be *specific*. "I want to walk" isn't a specific goal. But if you say, "I will to walk 30 minutes every day," that's a specific goal. At first, maybe you can't walk for 30 minutes at one time. Set some intermittent goals that will get you to that 30-minute goal. You also have to strive to reach at least a moderately brisk pace.

2. An exercise goal must be *achievable*. The average person is going to lose about one to two pounds a week. If you are extremely heavy, as I was, you may lose weight faster than that. In order to accelerate the weight loss, you have to exercise. In the beginning, set an achievable exercise goal.

3. The exercise goal must be *measurable*. That's the easy part. All you have to do is stand on a scale to see if you are reaching your weight goal. An exercise goal can be measured by using a pedometer or staking out a route of, say, one mile. Drive it in your car to measure the distance, then park the car and get walking.

If you are faithful in walking and eating healthy foods in small portions, you will lose weight. Then, stepping on the scale becomes a joyful experience as your weight creeps slowly downward.

A group of doctors who studied obese and overweight adults found that those who weighed themselves more often lost more weight and prevented more weight gain over a period of two years than those who weighed themselves less frequently. Contrary to the advice given in many popular weight-loss regimens, this study suggests that at least some people can benefit from the accountability brought on by daily weigh-ins. Potential advantages of daily weighing include the recognition of slow patterns of weight gain that may not be immediately apparent and the chance to modify lifestyle habits before the total weight gain becomes extreme and difficult to control.

One caveat: Because your weight fluctuates from day to day, daily weighing can lead to discouragement and potential diet sabotage if you see a higher number from one day to the next. Most diet experts believe that a weekly or even a monthly weigh-in is a more accurate reflection of weight control progress. I prefer the once-a-week weigh-in.

Your personality will likely play a role in deciding how often to weigh yourself. If you're easily discouraged, daily weighing might cause you to give up your attempts if you don't see rapid progress. On the other hand, if you crave control and feedback, daily weighing might satisfy more of your needs and fuel your motivation. Whatever weigh-in frequency you choose, keep these tips in mind when stepping on the scale:

1. Weighing yourself first thing in the morning is usually best. Because of variations in food and fluid consumption, we often "gain" different amounts of weight throughout the day.

2. If you're weighing frequently, remember that daily fluctuations in weight are common. Just because you're heavier today than yesterday doesn't mean your weight-control program isn't working. Don't become a slave to the numbers.

3. Monthly variations in weight are also common in menstruating women.

4. "Plateaus" in weight loss aren't necessarily bad. If you're exercising a lot, your weight may remain constant for a time as you build muscle, even though you're still decreasing your body fat content and getting healthier.

5. Finally, cues other than the numbers on the scale are equally important. How do you feel? Are your clothes getting looser or tighter? Do you feel stronger, healthier, leaner? Your own perceptions can be the most valuable tool to help you track your weight-control progress.

A Bod4God Close-Up

Pete Frenquelle
Lost 130 pounds

Before	After

I've gained and lost weight almost my entire life. I didn't gain it all at once. It was slow coming on. My eating habits led to gaining about a pound a month—12 pounds a year—but I did it for more than 10 years. That adds up to more than 120 pounds. When I was about 240 pounds, I really started feeling my weight. I gradually went on to 270, 300 and, finally, 350 pounds. At that point I could barely walk from my car to the church door. Sometimes I'd lose some weight, but then I regained even more than I had lost. It was three steps forward in weight gain and one step back in weight loss. I never really made any progress in losing weight. I hated looking in the mirror at what I had become.

For most of my adult life I've lived in either Florida or Virginia. When I moved back to Northern Virginia in 2008, to restore my career, a friend told me about Capital Baptist Church and its weight-loss program. I knew I needed to lose weight, so I decided to check out the church. In the beginning, I only came on Sunday nights for the weight-loss program.

In the past, I had always tried to lose weight on my own. But this program was completely different from anything I'd ever done before. For one thing, I'd never dedicated my weight problem to God. Additionally, I had always chosen unsustainable methods, saying something like "No restaurants . . . ever." Of course, I couldn't keep that promise. Bod4God is a lifestyle change. It encourages overweight people to make small changes for life. For example, I had gained a lot of weight by drinking sugared colas. I don't like diet colas, and it's a long way from sugared cola to water. I had to find an immediate small change. So if I had a soft drink urge, I drank club soda, sometimes mixed with fruit juice.

Some other small changes for life that I have made are:

- Smaller meals; more frequent meals
- Switching from white bread to whole-grain bread
- Eating breakfast to get my metabolism going
- My largest meal of the day is lunch, not dinner
- Dinner is a small meal, typically a salad or sandwich on whole grain bread
- I'm finished eating for the day by 6:00 or 6:30 in the evening
- Little increases in walking and moving throughout the day

As far as exercise, what I've learned is that the principles of momentum apply, both negatively and positively. The more weight you gain, the more you hate to move. The more you hate to move, the more weight you gain. Conversely, the more weight you lose, the more you want to move. The more you move, the more weight you lose.

This program is not a diet—you are learning principles and techniques that will set the course permanently for a healthier lifestyle. Anyone can make changes for one or two weeks, but you will eventually hit a plateau in your weight loss. Don't get discouraged. If you stick with the program, when you get past week four or five you will lose weight again. In high school we had something called "senior-itis." It meant that seniors coasted through the last part of their senior year and didn't try very hard to accomplish anything. We can't have "senior-itis" in our weight-loss program and expect to finish well. With God's help, I overcame my weight-loss plateau at weeks three and four and went on to finish strongly in week 10.

There is a parable in the Bible that struck me deeply because it was how I'd lived so much of my life. It's the parable of the seeds that come up quickly and are withered by the sun soon thereafter. When it came to long-term goals, I had a pattern of starting something and then abandoning it as soon as I encountered an obstacle. I finally made a decision to get one thing squared away in my life before I went to work on other areas of concern. I decided to start with my weight. Now that I've lost weight, I don't have that obstacle hindering other parts of my life. I can go on to accomplish other goals. I've found, though, that one has to have faith for the strength to overcome obstacles and the perseverance to finish well.

A huge factor in weight loss for me was team accountability. I joined a team. I met Eric Larsen. He was such an inspiration. Eric had lost 100 pounds in one year. I decided I'd like to do the same. Eric and I are now good friends. He has become one of my mentors as well. Eric had led the winning team in the competition prior to my joining and, in a subsequent competition, I wanted to do the same with the team I led. Our team strictly followed the Bod4God guideline. At the end of the Fall 2008 competition, my team won and had four of the top 10 losers.

The team meeting is essentially a small group Bible study with a healthy lifestyle theme. Prayer is at the core of everything we do. However, there are unique aspects of a Bod4God small group. Everyone picks a nickname. Mine is "Persistent Pete." The team also picks a name using a fruit or vegetable. Our name was the "Re-Formed Couch Potatoes."

Also, while each team differs in style, all teams adhere to certain core principles of Bod4God. First of all, we have a confidentiality rule. We need to be able to speak freely about problems in our lives that may be fueling our unhealthy eating habits. When participants arrive, they usually have already weighed in and are ready to discuss the evening's topic. We begin the meeting in prayer. There is also a Scripture verse that sets the tone for the discussion. Then we share successes and challenges we have had during the week and we report on small changes we have made in eating and exercise. Next, we discuss the questions in the Bod4God Victory Guide.

We have one hard and fast rule other than confidentiality, and that is that if you haven't done the work in the Victory Guide, you can't talk in the meeting. Since the weekly reading assignments are not very long, usually everyone has done their homework. Then we share a small change that we have made the previous week. Sometimes there is a "book of the week" suggestion for a deeper understanding of a particular health-related topic. If there is time, members share what they are facing in the next week and how they plan to successfully meet the challenge. We then close in prayer.

There are a lot of good people in the program and it starts at the top with Pastor Reynolds. I still have some weight to lose, but my challenge is not just about weight loss anymore. It is now about fitness. I've gone from not being able to get from the car to the church door to planning to walk in a 5K the church sponsors. I still can't run, but I can walk!

The man lying on the mat by the pool of Bethesda (see John 5) had been there for 38 years when Jesus healed him. I was 38 years old when I started the Bod4God program. Jesus changed that man's life, and He has changed mine too. I am thankful.

Small Steps to Life Ideas

What Do You Need to Know About H₂O?

Drinking a pint of water will increase metabolism for about a half-hour, causing the body to burn about 25 calories. Researchers believe that the increase in metabolism comes from warming the water in the stomach. That means that if you drink a pint of water before a meal, you will rev up your metabolism as well as make your stomach feel full. It will help you eat less and burn more when you do eat your meal. Let's look at a couple more changes you can make in eating and exercise.

Small Food Steps

How about a great recipe to encourage your healthy eating? This one is a healthy wrap. Wraps are great because they are creative, individual and versatile. For a great wrap, create a combination of the following ingredients:

1. Tortillas (whole-wheat, tomato, spinach, roasted garlic); lean meat (turkey, roast beef, roasted chicken, grilled chicken, tuna, spicy shrimp, even leftover steak)
2. Salad greens or vegetables (Lettuce, olives, salsa)
3. Lowfat cheese (cheddar, jalapeño jack, provolone)
4. Lowfat dressing (ranch, chipotle ranch blue cheese, balsamic vinaigrette)

Spread salad dressing on the tortilla. (You might want to steam, microwave or heat the tortilla so that it becomes soft for easy rolling.) Layer lean meat, cheese and vegetables on the tortilla and then roll tightly. Cut and serve with a lowfat side dish (vinegar slaw, roasted vegetable salad or a lowfat grain salad). (Recipe courtesy of Chef Bobby Vickers, CEC, CCA, CFBE.)

Small Exercise Steps

There are a number of small exercise steps given in this chapter already, but let's add one more: Leg lifts while sitting at the computer. Do five reps, two to three times a day.

Small Steps to Life Record

What "Skinny Things" Will You Do This Week?

Fill out this chart each week by indicating: (1) What you will do to eat less to live; (2) What you will do to exercise more to live; and (3) What average daily ounces of water you will drink. Pick only a few things, and stick with them. Remember that weight loss and maintenance requires you to *eat less* and *exercise more*.

Sun.	
Mon.	
Tues.	
Wed.	
Thurs.	
Fri.	
Sat.	

Bod4God Victory Guide

To apply the information in this chapter to your life, work through the Victory Guide. It will equip you to practice the four keys to weight loss. Big losers make the Victory Guide a high priority. Record this week's weight change on "My Progress Report" located in appendix A.

Week Eight: *E* Is for Exercise

Memory Verse

"Therefore, whether you eat or drink, or whatever you do, do all to the glory of God" (1 Cor. 10:31).

Reflection/Application Questions

1. First Corinthians 10:31 gives the basic principle by which believers are to determine their conduct. Everything we do must honor God. That is to be our motivation. In your opinion, how does a person exercise to the glory of God?

   _____

   _____

   _____

   _____

   _____

   _____

   _____

2. How would you describe your past exercise habits? Do they honor God? Explain.

   _____

   _____

   _____

   _____

   _____

   _____

   _____

3. In what ways are you physically active on a daily basis? What is your weekly exercise routine? Write your daily activity in the chart below.

Sun.	
Mon.	
Tues.	
Wed.	
Thurs.	
Fri.	
Sat.	

4. In 1 Timothy 4:8, Paul's emphasis is on godliness rather than physical exercise. Note that Paul is not downgrading the importance of physical exercise, just that he is emphasizing godliness. You cannot ignore one (godliness) to pursue the other (healthy body). Are you as concerned about godliness as you are about physical exercise?

_____

_____

_____

_____

_____

5. In what ways are you exercising yourself to become more godly?

_____

_____

_____

_____

_____

6. As I mentioned in this chapter, you have to set goals of output to achieve your goals of input. My output goal was to lose 100 pounds, while my input goals were all of the "Small Steps to Life" I

developed to meet the output goal of major weight loss. What is
your output goal?

_____

_____

_____

_____

_____

7. Have you written this goal down? If so, where will you post it so you
    can see it on a daily basis?

_____

_____

_____

_____

_____

8. What input goals will you need to put in place to help you achieve
    your output goal?

_____

_____

_____

_____

_____

9. Temptation will come. What are some of the greatest temptations
    you face in your struggle to become healthy? What are you doing to
    handle those difficult times?

_____

_____

_____

_____

_____

My Bod4God Journal

Teach me, O Lord, the way of Your statutes, and I shall keep it to the end.
PSALM 119:33

Record what God is telling you to do this week to apply the four keys to a better body.

Dedication: Honoring God with My Body

_____
_____
_____
_____
_____

Inspiration: Motivating Myself for Change

_____
_____
_____
_____
_____

Eat and Exercise: Managing My Habits

_____
_____
_____
_____

Team: Building My Circle of Support

_____
_____
_____
_____

T Is for Team:
A Personal Challenge

Restore to me the joy of Your salvation, and uphold me by Your generous Spirit.
PSALM 51:12

Let's talk some more about obesity. Physicians, weight trainers and other health personnel are talking more about Body Mass Index (BMI) than they are the actual pounds that show up on the scale as gained or lost. That's because muscle is heavier than fat, and the scale may be standing still if you are increasing muscle by exercising. Even though you may weigh the same, it could be that you are replacing fat with muscle. That's good, because muscle burns fat. The more muscle to fat ratio in your body, the higher your fat-burning metabolism. That's why men often have an advantage over women in their ability to lose weight more quickly. Women can even out that advantage by adding strength training to their aerobic exercise.

Everyone needs to know his or her BMI, and it is easy to calculate. There are a number of BMI calculators on the web. The one I like best is by the Department of Health and Human Services/National Institutes of Health at http://www.nhlbisupport.com/bmi/bmicalc.htm. There, you can enter your height and weight and in an instant know what your BMI is. If your BMI is between 25 and 29, you are overweight. If it is more than 30, you are obese. There is other valuable information on this website about the risks of being overweight or obese. There are ideas for helping you deal with your problem and even healthful recipes.

"Obesity" becomes "morbid obesity" when it significantly increases the risk of one or more obesity-related health conditions or serious

37 - 23

diseases (also known as co-morbidities). Morbid obesity—sometimes called "clinically severe obesity"—is defined as being 100 pounds or more over ideal body weight, or having a BMI of 40 or higher.[1]

The Learning Channel (TLC) recently aired a tragic program about a man named John Keitz. John weighed 750 pounds at the time the show began recording his journey. He had not left his bed in seven years because his legs simply could not handle the weight of his massive body. He could not even turn over in bed by himself. His wife and sister tried to care for him, but at last he was placed in a facility that attempts to help the morbidly obese. John was diabetic and had other multiple health problems as a direct result of his weight. Unfortunately, it was too late. John developed septic shock resulting from open sores on his skin caused by the pressure of his flesh against the bed and his extreme weight. He died at the age of 39.

John, like myself, weighed more than 100 pounds in first grade. Unlike me, he did not play sports, and there is no evidence that he ever had an encounter with God about caring for his body, like I did. I realize that if God had not intervened in my life, I could have been John. I could be gone by now.

A second story on TLC documented another obese person—a 627-pound woman named Jackie. She, too, was bedridden, but with great effort she could still turn herself. She opted for gastric bypass surgery. The procedure required a huge incision so surgeons could repair a massive hernia Jackie's body had developed and which had caused a large portion of her internal organs to be displaced.

Something went awry in Jackie's surgery and condition, and instead of reducing the amount of food she could take in—one ounce in the beginning and expanding to half a cup later on—Jackie couldn't keep anything down. Did she lose weight? Oh, yes, the weight fell off her, but she was also not getting any nutrients to her system. The decision was made to insert a feeding tube that she had for many months. She is still struggling to overcome both her obesity and the results of the surgery.

Why am I telling you these stories? Because I want you to face the fact that you may be either overweight and headed toward obesity or you may even be obese and headed toward morbid obesity and certain death as a direct result. I am pleading with you to do something now—today—about your weight and unhealthy eating habits. Face reality and save your own life.

One more thing; John, whose story was told on TLC, had stashes of chips and cookies hidden in his room at the clinic. Someone had to be bringing this junk food to him because he was unable to go get it himself. Perhaps you are not the one with the weight problem; perhaps you are the enabler who is helping your loved one stay obese. It's time for both of you to get honest and face the truth.

Obesity Is a Big Problem

Obesity has reached epidemic proportions in the United States. Approximately 66 percent of people here are considered overweight or obese (with a BMI of greater than or equal to 25) and 32 percent—72 million Americans—can be diagnosed as obese (with a BMI greater than or equal to 30). More than one million people are "super obese," with a BMI of 50 or more.[2] This trend toward obesity has been rapidly escalating for the last 10 to 15 years. The worst offenders are in Middle America and the southeastern part of the country.

Some of the "fattest cities" in the U.S., according to *Forbes* magazine, include Memphis, Tennessee, with 34 percent obesity; Birmingham, Alabama, and San Antonio, Texas, with 31 percent; and Riverside, California, and Detroit, Michigan, at 30 percent obesity. Washington, D.C., is number one for having the fattest kids in the nation. One in four children between the ages of 10 and 17 years old, living there, are obese.[3] Are you shocked? You should be.

What's really sad is that this epidemic is preventable. Obesity is the most common preventable cause of death second only to smoking. According to the National Institutes of Health, it is the major cause of 30 medical conditions that are costing our society $92.6 billion annually.[4] One of the big conditions is cardiovascular disease (CVD). Seventy percent of CVD is caused by obesity, along with high blood pressure, elevated cholesterol and triglycerides.[5] Eighty percent of Type II diabetes, which can lead to blindness, kidney failure and vascular disease, with limb amputations, is caused by obesity.[6] Arthritis is linked to obesity, with two times the risk of developing arthritis at a BMI of 30, and four times the risk at 40 BMI.[7]

Digestive problems such as gallstones, cirrhosis, sleep apnea and a multitude of other physical conditions, including the presence of excess body and facial hair are exacerbated by obesity. Half of breast cancers and colon cancer are related to obesity.[8] Endometrial cancer is four times as common in the obese, along with stomach and esophageal cancer.[9]

Why would any thinking person not do something about his or her obesity once these facts are presented? Is that super-sized meal, that four-layer chocolate cake and endless bowls of ice cream really worth your health? On the other hand, losing weight can cause you to live longer, have more energy, feel better, save money on both medical and pharmacy costs and honor the Lord by taking care of the body He has given you.

Ask God to Be Your Personal Trainer

"But Pastor Steve," I hear you whine, "I don't have anyone to work with. I don't have a team. I can't do this by myself." Sorry, friend, but that dog don't hunt. There are no excuses for not caring for your own body, the beautiful, finely tuned machine God gave you as your place of residence on earth. If you don't have anyone to work with, you are going to have to do it alone. Is it hard? Yes. Is it harder than working with a team to lose weight? Probably. But it can be done. I lost 70 pounds before we ever established the Losing to Live competitions. If I can do it, you can too.

That said, you have to have support for your weight-loss program even if you are doing it on your own. First, you have to get God on your team. I have a sneaking hunch that He has been hanging around waiting for you to get to this place. He wants your body to be all it can be. He has plans for you and for your life. He wants to help you.

Let's think of doing it alone as a team of one plus One—the second One being God Almighty who is able to do "above all that we ask or think" (Eph. 3:20). Here are some Scriptures to help you through those tough times.

Put God on Your Team

Taste and see that the LORD is good; blessed is the man who trusts in Him! (Ps. 34:8).

Blessed are those who hunger and thirst for righteousness, for they shall be filled (Matt. 5:6).

Live a Full Life in God

So I became great and excelled more than all who were before me in Jerusalem. Also, my wisdom remained with me. Whatever my eyes desired I did not keep from them. I did not withhold my heart from any pleasure. For my heart rejoiced in all my labor; and this was my reward from all my labor. Then I looked on all the works that my hands had done and on the labor in which I had toiled; and indeed all was vanity and grasping for the wind. There was no profit under the sun (Eccles. 2:9-11).

Rely on God for the Victory

If you faint in the day of adversity, your strength is small (Prov.24:10).

I am the vine, you are the branches. He who abides in Me, and I in him, bears much fruit; for without Me you can do nothing (John 15:5).

Pray Regularly

Call to Me, and I will answer you, and show you great and mighty things, which you do not know (Jer. 33:3).

Men always ought to pray and not lose heart (Luke 18:1).

Be Consistent in Daily Bible Reading

I have not departed from the commandment of His lips; I have treasured the words of His mouth more than my necessary food (Job 23:12).

Your words were found, and I ate them, and Your word was to me the joy and rejoicing of my heart; for I am called by Your name, O LORD God of hosts (Jer. 15:16).

Man shall not live by bread alone, but by every word that proceeds from the mouth of God (Matt. 4:4).

Attend Church Weekly and Participate in Church Activities

I was glad when they said to me, "Let us go into the house of the LORD" (Ps. 122:1).

Let us consider one another in order to stir up love and good works, not forsaking the assembling of ourselves together, as is the manner of some, but exhorting one another, and so much the more as you see the Day approaching (Heb. 10:24-25).

The whole body, joined and knit together by what every joint supplies, according to the effective working by which every part does its share, causes growth of the body for the edifying of itself in love (Eph. 4:16).

Choose a Top-Notch Team

The Bible says, "He who walks with wise men will be wise, but the companion of fools will be destroyed" (Prov. 13:20). I had to choose wise people to be part of my team. I had to find people who would come alongside me as Aaron and Hur did for Moses, recorded in Exodus 17:12. Every time Moses held up his hands and stood for God, his team won the war. But when he dropped his hands because his arms were heavy, the team lost. Aaron and Hur came alongside to hold up his arms. Your team is crucial for winning the war on obesity. Who is going to hold up your hands?

I intentionally sought out people who could help me. There were three kinds of people I chose for my team:

People Who Will Educate You

I chose students of health. I read. I studied. I talked to people who had also lost weight. But first and foremost, I talked to my doctor. You really must make a point to see a doctor before you begin any eating and exercise changes. My doctor played a major role in my weight loss and was always there to ask me how I was doing with my eating and exercising. For a long time I didn't have any good news to report to him. I was a diabetic, and I was supposed to see the doctor frequently. I didn't go because I didn't want him to tell me again and again what I should be doing and wasn't. Maybe you can relate to this. My doctor never backed down. He just kept asking. When I started exercising, he didn't tell me I was doing well to exercise three times a week. He said, "You eat every day, why don't you exercise every day?" I had to acknowledge he made a good point.

Authors are among the people who can educate you. Read books, articles, and web pages written by people who can help you learn about good health. There is a huge amount of information available today, so there is no excuse for being ignorant about your health. "But books and magazines cost so much," I hear you protest. Think of this educational material as an investment in your own body. You are worth it! If you truly can't afford to own some books, use the public library. You'll find plenty there to educate your mind about good health.

People Who Will Encourage You

Find some people who will encourage you. You need to have role models. As I said earlier, Mike Huckabee, who has a show on Fox News Network and is the former governor of Arkansas is my role model. I look to him as a great example. I've seen his life, and I've read his book on how he lost weight.

I'm also encouraged when I see all the people at Capital Baptist Church who have lost weight. I know this program—this lifestyle change—works, because I've seen it in action. If I were ever discouraged, all I'd have to do is sit down with Rich or Eric or any of the others and say, "Tell me your weight-loss story again," and I'd be encouraged to go on. It is truly amazing what these participants, along with God's help, have done about getting their bodies back to health.

People Who Will Equip You

Finally, we all need people who will equip us—those who can show us how to do what we've purposed to do. Many people are the same as I was. They don't exercise. I think it would be great to have a personal trainer working with me on a regular basis, but I don't. However, the first time I went to the gym to exercise, a personal trainer took me around to show me the machines. He explained how to use each piece of equipment at the gym without injuring myself and told me what each piece of equipment would do to help me. He taught me how to build my endurance on each apparatus.

That personal trainer had lost more than 100 pounds himself. He was the one who introduced me to the CLIF BAR.™ It is an organic bar that has about 12 grams of protein, 6 grams of fat, 5 grams of fiber and about 260 calories. I eat one every morning. I am thankful that my trainer not only equipped me to work on the machines, but he also told me about a nutritional item that has been a great help to me.

One other equipping help is the Body & Soul exercise program held at our church, which I mentioned earlier in the book. Perhaps joining such a program would work better for you than a gym workout. You have to find people and programs that can equip you for the long battle of losing weight. The good news is that after only a few days of exercise, you will begin to feel better than you have in a long time. That's something to look forward to right now.

A Team of Relationships

Of course, most important in my weight loss was that God and I were on the same side of the fence. In addition, I realized that I had to get my relationships across that fence too. I had to talk to my wife and kids and tell them what I was trying to do. I had to talk to my coworkers. I had to talk to my friends. I even had to talk to my mother. I couldn't have any of them sabotaging my plans for weight loss. You know, comments such as, "Just one piece of pie. You deserve it. You've worked so hard this week. And besides, I made it just for you."

I had to build a circle of support for my newfound journey to a healthy lifestyle. I had to ask for help. And that's not always easy for guys to do. I've learned that when a couple has a marriage problem, it's usually the wife who calls me for help. Guys, unfortunately, are embarrassed to ask for help. But, guys—I'm talking to you now, we have to get over it if we're going to get the support we need for our weight-loss program.

If you are planning to lose weight without the benefit of a team, first enlist God's help and then find yourself a partner. There is probably at least one other person in your circle of church friends who wants to lose weight too. Or maybe there's someone at your workplace. Set up a time when you email each other, get together or talk on the phone about your victories or snags. Get a prayer partner to commit to praying for you on a daily basis. Share your successes with all your contacts and reward yourself . . . but not with food.

Let's go back to the Mayo Clinic website one more time to see what they say about doing it alone on a weight-loss program. Here are six strategies for success:

1. *Make a commitment.* Only you can make the commitment to treat your body better. External pressure from the people closest to you may scuttle your efforts to lose weight. You have to decide to lose weight to please yourself. It's a good idea to clear up any other major issues in your life so that you aren't distracted by them as you launch your weight-loss program.

2. *Get emotional support.* Pick people who want what's best for you and will encourage you. Find people who will listen to your concerns and feelings and who are willing to exercise with you for a healthier lifestyle.

3. *Set a realistic goal.* Aim to lose one to two pounds a week. You'll have to burn 500 to 1,000 more calories than you take in each day to accomplish this goal. Make your goals

"process goals," such as exercising regularly, rather than "outcome goals," such as losing 50 pounds. Change your lifestyle by making Small Steps to Life.

4. *Learn to enjoy healthier foods.* Eat more plant-based foods such as fruit, vegetables and whole grains. Strive for variety to help you achieve your goals without giving up taste or nutrition.

5. *Get active, stay active.* Cutting 500 calories from your daily diet can help you lose about a pound a week. But, if you add a 45- to 60-minute brisk walk four days a week, you will double your rate of weight loss. The goal of exercise is to burn calories. Even though regularly scheduled aerobic exercise is best for losing fat, any extra movement helps burn calories. Think about ways you can increase your physical activity throughout the day.

6. *Change your lifestyle* rather than considering yourself on a diet for a certain period of time. You have to make lifestyle changes that will remain in place all the way to the end of your life.

Dealing with Those Who Doubt

Those who doubt are everywhere. And as soon as you get serious about losing weight, they come out of the woodwork and start saying things like: "So how many times have you been on a diet before?" and "Yoo-hoo, everybody, Pastor Steve's gonna get skinny. What do ya think about that? Think he can do it?" I'm not sure if it's jealousy that drives this kind of talk, or an attitude or what. If you've been up and down in your weight as I have, maybe these folks really don't believe you can change. Come to think of it, why would they believe that this time will be different?

You just can't let them get to you. You have to realize it took you a while to get into this overweight situation and it's going to take a while to get out. People will begin to believe you are serious and will help you when they see you sticking to your Small Steps to Life and that you are beginning to lose weight.

Spend some time reading the story of Daniel and think about the food choice he made. The king wanted Daniel to eat the richest foods the kingdom had to offer. He wanted Daniel to be healthy and thought that was the way to ensure his health. But Daniel knew something the king didn't. He knew the diet the king proposed would damage his health both physically and spiritually. Here's the story from *THE MESSAGE:*

> But Daniel determined that he would not defile himself by eating the king's food or drinking his wine, so he asked the head of the palace staff to exempt him from the royal diet. The head of the palace staff, by God's grace, liked Daniel, but he warned him, "I'm afraid of what my master the king will do. He is the one who assigned this diet and if he sees that you are not as healthy as the rest, he'll have my head!"
>
> But Daniel appealed to a steward who had been assigned by the head of the palace staff to be in charge of Daniel, Hananiah, Mishael, and Azariah: "Try us out for ten days on a simple diet of vegetables and water. Then compare us with the young men who eat from the royal menu. Make your decision on the basis of what you see."
>
> The steward agreed to do it and fed them vegetables and water for ten days. At the end of the ten days they looked better and more robust than all the others who had been eating from the royal menu. So the steward continued to exempt them from the royal menu of food and drink and served them only vegetables (Dan. 1:8-16).

The king represented someone negative in Daniel's life, and Daniel had to resolve to stick by his decision not to eat from the king's table. It worked. You, too, are going to have to deal with negative people, most of whom don't mean to be negative, but they truly can sabotage your plan. Also notice that in just 10 days Daniel saw some results from healthy eating, and you can too!

What to Do About the Workplace

If ever there is a place to scuttle your weight-loss program, it is the workplace. Think about it. First, there are all the parties that happen during work hours. There are birthday parties, wedding and baby showers, retirement and welcoming parties, Christmas parties and on and on it goes. Every one of them is a trap to set you back days in your efforts to eat healthy. Then there are the lunches and dinners out entertaining guests, and business trips on an all-expense-paid business credit card that just begs you to spend money on a "really great" meal since the company is paying for it. The company may be paying money for the meal, but who is really paying for overeating and eating the wrong things? You are. If entertaining and eating out is a continuing lifestyle for you, you are probably wearing the result of workplace sabotage right around your middle.

What can you do about this serious problem in your health-conscious life? One thing you can do is watch what the skinny people at your company do. Do they load up on carbs at the event? Do they even eat? When eating out, do they eat the whole meal with appetizers included, or do they push back the plate when they've eaten half or less of the meal? Do they ask for a doggie bag? You can learn a lot from observing them.

Acknowledge that no one is forcing you to eat all the cookies, cakes, ice cream and candy that show up at your workplace. You won't get your pay docked if you don't eat them. No one will twist your arm if you pass them by. Truly, most people won't pay any attention to whether you are eating the desserts or not. Be honest and admit that you are eating the junk food because you made a decision to eat it. You want it. Acknowledging that you have a problem is the first step to overcoming it.

Let's think of some ways to deal with this workplace problem.

- One thing you can do is make a game of the event to see how little you can eat and not have anyone notice.

- Take a small piece of cake or a cookie on a plate. Carry the plate around with you and keep talking to everyone. Don't eat what's on the plate, just carry it around. It will keep others from refilling your plate.

- Even better is to carry around a glass of punch, soft drink or cup of coffee. You don't have to drink it, just carry it around and when asked if you've had the dessert just say, "I'm fine with this," and indicate the drink.

- Think about what the purpose of the event is. Usually it is to honor someone. So instead of eating, spend the time talking to the honoree and other guests. It will make you very popular as a guest.

- Leave as quickly as you can and reduce the temptation to eat by simply walking away from it.

- Don't volunteer to help clean up unless you have been assigned that task. There is too much temptation to nibble the leftovers.

- If you are planning the party, be sure to include some snack trays with veggies and fruit with lowfat and/or sugar-free dips and dressings for yourself and the others who are eating healthy as well.

- Eat a small healthy snack before you go to the event. A handful of almonds is a good choice.

- Get active. Part of the problem of weight gain at the office is the inactivity of sitting behind a desk all day. There are some great exercises you can do right at your desk. Set a timer to remind you to do these simple exercises:

  1. For your tummy: Sit tall and straighten the spine. Then clench the abdominal muscles as tightly as possible, pulling your bellybutton back toward the spine. Hold for one to five seconds and repeat 20 times. Do at least three times daily.

2. For your thighs: While seated with knees together, imagine someone's pulling them apart and it's your job to keep them together by squeezing your inner thigh muscles in one-second pulses. Do this at least three times daily.

3. For your backside: Start to stand up, with heels digging into the ground to contract the backside muscles, but pause a beat about three-quarters of the way through the standing motion. Sit back down, and then, finally stand up as you normally would. It's a great way to get exercise without even breaking a sweat.

- Better yet, go for a walk on your lunch break. Just bring a pair of walking shoes and keep them under your desk.

I hope you see now that even if you don't have a group competition and an established group to help you, you can still be a team of one and ask God to join you in this very important battle for your body and your future. He is just waiting for you to ask for His help, and He will bring resources to you of which you have never dreamed.

Notes
1. Information taken from the Highland Hospital website, University of Rochester Medical Center, www.urmc.rochester.edu/hh/.
2. "Prevalence of Overweight and Obesity Among Adults: United States, 2003-2004," National Center for Health Statistics, April 2006. http://www.cdc.gov/nchs/products/pubs/pubd/hestats/overweight/overwght_adult_03.htm.
3. Rebecca Ruiz, "America's Most Obese Cities," *Forbes,* November 26, 2007. http://www.forbes.com/2007/11/14/health-obesity-cities-forbeslife-cx_rr_1114obese.html.
4. "Statistics Related to Overweight and Obesity," National Institute of Diabetes and Kidney Diseases, May 2007. http://win.niddk.nih.gov/statistics/index.htm.
5. Kadence Buchanan, "The Epidemic of Obesity," The Free Library, 2007. http://www.thefreelibrary.com/The+Epidemic+of+Obesity-a01073781449.
6. "Statistics Related to Overweight and Obesity," National Institute of Diabetes and Kidney Diseases, May 2007.

7. Chetna Mehrota, MPH, OTR, Timothy S. Naimi, MD, MPH, Mary Serdula, MD, MPH, et al, "Arthritis, Body Mass Index, and Professional Advice to Lose Weight: Implications for Clinical Medicine and Public Health," *American Journal of Preventive Medicine,* July 2004, vol. 27, no. 1, pp. 16-21. http://www.ajpm-online.net/article/S0749-3797(04)00051-0/abstract.

8. T.G. Key, P.N. Appleby, G.K. Reeves, et al, "An Overview on the Link Between Cancer and Obesity," *Journal of the National Cancer Institute,* 2003, vol. 95, no. 16, pp. 1218-1226. http://74.125.113.132/search?q=cache:v039N2FgUU4J:www.eatrightiowa.org/membersonly/marketingfiles/CCC.press%2520release%2520abbreviated.doc+50+percent+breast+cancer+colon+cancer+obesity&cd=3&hl=en&ct=clnk&gl=us&client=firefox-a.

9. Rudolf Kaaks, Annekatrin Lukanova and Mindy S. Kurzer, "Obesity, Endogenous Hormones, and Endometrial Cancer Risk," *Cancer Epidemiology Biomarkers and Prevention,* December 2002, vol. 11, pp. 1531-1543. http://cebp.aacrjournals.org/cgi/content/full/11/12/1531.

Before

After

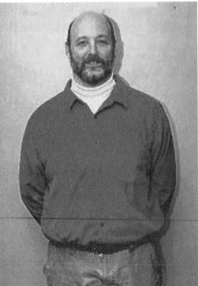

Before

After

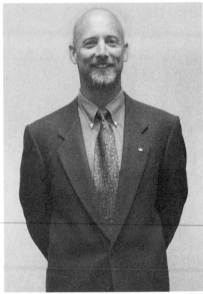

A Bod4God Close-Up

Robert and Caroline Murphy
Robert: lost 34 pounds
Caroline: lost 39 pounds

Caroline and Robert Murphy both took part in a Losing to Live competition. While the competition was important to them, Caroline says that what really stuck out in her mind was when Pastor Steve talked about team and how important a team is to success in weight loss. "My strongest support system is my family," Caroline says. "They are my team."

Robert says, "I joined the competition to encourage my wife and do it with her." After Robert and Caroline began to exercise, their two teenage boys began to come with them to exercise in the Body & Soul program. The program has since had many side benefits for the family besides exercise and weight loss. Caroline says, "Since joining the program, we pray more together, and we read more together. My husband has us memorizing the book of James together. It is a good foundation for our kids."

Small Steps to Life Ideas

Remember, Rome wasn't built in a day, and neither will your new body be built in a day or even a week or month. But little by little you will lay a new foundation for your new body, and little by little you will build new eating and exercise habits on that foundation; and one day, you'll look in the mirror at a new you. You can do this!

What Do You Need to Know About H_2O?

Pastor Steve starts drinking a lot of water first thing in the morning and drinks water all day long as his main beverage. He may vary what he drinks in the evening. He also eats lots fruits and vegetables that have a high water content.

Small Food Steps

Eat breakfast. Eating breakfast gets your metabolism going for the day. That gives you more energy. If you skip breakfast, you set yourself up to snack during the morning, often on high-fat foods (donuts and sweet rolls). Missing breakfast can also cause you to eat too much food later in the day at other meals.

- Eating breakfast every day may reduce the risk for obesity and insulin resistance syndrome—an early sign of developing diabetes—by as much as 35 to 50 percent, according to a study presented at a recent American Heart Association conference.

- Eat whole-grain cereal. Look for cereals that list whole grain or bran as their first ingredient and contain at least 2 grams of dietary fiber per serving. Bran cereal and oatmeal contain at least 7 grams per serving, or about 25 percent of the recommended daily intake. Fiber One cereal contains 15 grams of fiber for a half cup.

- No time is not an excuse. Here's a quick way to make oatmeal—a great breakfast cereal. Pour one cup of water in a good-sized microwavable bowl (the cereal bubbles up when cooking). Add ½ cup of old-fashioned oats (steel cut are the best). Just don't use instant as they turn into something resembling wallpaper paste. Add a tablespoon of raisins or other dried fruit. You can add cinnamon, nutmeg or maple flavoring (not maple syrup). Microwave four minutes. You can add a few almonds, skim milk or lowfat soy milk. It doesn't get much faster than that for a quick, hot, nourishing breakfast.

- If cereal is not for you first thing in the morning, make a fruit smoothie with yogurt. Or have lowfat cheese and whole-grain crackers. Peanut butter spread on whole-wheat toast or a bagel fills you up.

- Search the fridge for leftovers that are tasty and nutritious. Who says you can't eat stir-fry in the morning, or a slice of whole-wheat vegetarian pizza?!

Small Exercise Steps

If you work at a desk, try the exercises given on pages 185-186. Some call these "deskercises." These days, many exercise programs offer chair options.

- Buy an aerobic or other kind of exercise CD and begin working out with it. You don't have to spend a lot of money. You can find many such tapes and CDs in thrift shops and places that resell CDs.

- Your local library offers all sorts of free health information, including exercise books.

Small Steps to Life Record

What "Skinny Things" Will You Do this Week?

Fill out this chart each week by indicating: (1) What you will do to eat less to live, (2) What you will do to exercise more to live, and (3) What average daily ounces of water you will drink. Pick only a few things, and stick with them. Remember that weight loss and maintenance requires you to *eat less* and *exercise more*.

Sun.	
Mon.	
Tues.	
Wed.	
Thurs.	
Fri.	
Sat.	

Bod4God Victory Guide

To apply the information in this chapter to your life, work through the Victory Guide. It will equip you to practice the four keys to weight loss. Big losers make the Victory Guide a high priority. Record this week's weight change on "My Progress Report" located in appendix A.

Week Nine: *T* Is for Team: A Personal Challenge

Memory Verse
"Restore to me the joy of Your salvation, and uphold me by Your generous Spirit" (Ps. 51:12).

Reflection/Application Questions
1. In what way does Psalm 51:12 give you motivation in continuing with your Bod4God lifestyle plan?

   _____

   _____

   _____

   _____

   _____

2. Proverbs 13:20 says that if we want to be wise, we need to walk with wise people. Who should be part of your team? (Remember, there are people on my team I have never met personally, but they have educated, encouraged and equipped me.) Write the names of these people below.

   People who will educate you

   _____

   _____

   _____

   _____

   _____

People who will encourage you

_____

_____

_____

_____

_____

People who will equip you

_____

_____

_____

_____

_____

3. Can you identify someone who might be negative about your attempt to lose weight? What will you do to deal with that negativity?

_____

_____

_____

_____

_____

_____

_____

4. Read Matthew 18:15. What techniques does this Scripture offer as a way to handle negative people?

_____

_____

_____

_____

_____

_____

_____

5. Read Daniel 1. What techniques does this Scripture offer as a way to handle negative people?

_____

_____

_____

_____

_____

_____

_____

_____

6. What do you need to do to avoid temptation in your workplace?

_____

_____

_____

_____

_____

_____

_____

_____

_____

My Bod4God Journal

Teach me, O Lord, the way of Your statutes, and I shall keep it to the end.

PSALM 119:33

Record what God is telling you to do this week to apply the four keys to a better body.

Dedication: Honoring God with My Body

_____
_____
_____
_____
_____

Inspiration: Motivating Myself for Change

_____
_____
_____
_____
_____

Eat and Exercise: Managing My Habits

_____
_____
_____
_____

Team: Building My Circle of Support

_____
_____
_____
_____

T Is for Team:
A Group Competition

Two are better than one, because they have a good reward for their labor.
ECCLESIASTES 4:9

Why can't the local church be a place where people learn how to live healthy and lose weight? The Bible clearly commands Christians to have a Bod4God, and local churches must help people in this area. I've said it before, but it bears repeating—I'm not content to see only my own Bod4God plans achieved. I want to see a whole church—in fact entire churches—full of Bod4God losers. When I preached the "Bod4God: Four Keys to a Better Body" sermon series at Capital Baptist Church, my goal was to motivate our congregation to become the biggest group of losers in the United States. I would like to tell you about our first competition and how you can set up a competition in your church (see also appendix D).

I knew that a sermon series alone wasn't going to help people get to their weight goals. So, coinciding with the series, we launched the Losing to Live Weight Loss Competition as an opportunity to lose weight in a fun, supportive environment. It was a natural outflow of the "Team" key. I wanted to give others the same kind of team support and motivation I had received from my own group of encouragers.

What I found, after experiencing this competition, was that the 150 people who joined the competition—a large percentage of whom weren't members of our church—became my encouragement, motivation and inspiration. I felt as if they had come alongside me in making a difference for me, for themselves and for so many people all around them.

To open up the plan to those outside our congregation (as an outreach and a ministry to them), we advertised on local radio and with brochures and an announcement on the church's marquee. Our materials offered this invitation: "Don't try to lose weight by yourself. Join a team of losers at Capital Baptist Church."

With the media attention from the *Washington Post* and local and national (later, even international) TV, people came in droves to find out what would motivate a Baptist pastor to take such a personal interest in his congregation's physical health. Then, when Fox News' Neil Cavuto labeled me the "anti-fat pastor," it certainly got people's attention.

We kicked off our first competition on Sunday, January 14, 2007, with—of all things—an orientation luncheon. I shared the details of the competition and invited people to participate. A professional chef, and member of our church, prepared a beautiful (and delicious) healthy spread. Lots of vegetables and tasty salads along with a "wrap bar" that let participants choose healthy meats, cheeses and veggies to fold into their own soft tortilla wrappers.

The opening was a great rah-rah event, and dozens of people found themselves surprised that they were enjoying the healthy fare every bit as much as their old unhealthy choices. This was the first among countless successes experienced by participants, who lost a total of 1,310 pounds.

One of our Losing to Live participants, kindergarten teacher Peggy Ottenheimer, lost 24 pounds. She says, "I was on a lowfat diet for 10 years and didn't lose weight. I joined a gym and went for two years. Still no loss. It just wasn't happening." But Peggy is now successful, and she credits her success this time to being part of a Losing to Live team. "I needed a group to hold me accountable. It was a combination of things. First, I had to dedicate my weight to God, and then, I had to lose weight to God's glory. The team provided the extra oomph I needed—the accountability of our whole group—to lose weight.

What Happens at a Weekly Meeting

Each week during a competition, competitors have the opportunity to weigh in (in privacy, using a good scale) during each of our three Sunday morning services, as well as during our Sunday evening competition group meetings. Many prefer weighing in early in the day (before Sunday lunch or dinner), and that is fine with us.

At the big gathering in the church auditorium on Sunday evening, we open the session by announcing our weight-loss results and celebrating each team's achievements of the previous week. This is an inspiring time as the teams—each having chosen a fruit name (lemon and passion fruit) or a vegetable name (squash and rutabagas) to celebrate their total team weight-loss percentages. Individuals on the teams also compete to become one of the top 10 losers.

Input from Experts

After the cheerleading session, we invite experts to be speakers to the whole group. One week, for example, a board certified internal medicine physician in our congregation, Liz Berbano, might give us an update on the latest medical research on how to "fight back" against obesity. Another week the husband of one of our competitors (who is a certified internist) might come on a Sunday morning during weigh-in to offer baseline blood work (glucose and cholesterol) and take a blood pressure reading for the minimal fee of $15 to any competitor who wishes to participate.

Another week someone like Vivian Hutson, a registered dietician from our congregation, might be a guest speaker. Vivian has become key to our program, as she directs the weighing in of each participant week after week, offering encouragement and challenging them when needed. Vivian has a great story. She's been involved as a key player in creating our church's health ministry plan. Her training gives her a unique perspective to offer competitors, and the knowledge on how best to motivate them.

Vivian found the weigh-in times were great opportunities to get to know people and listen to their deeper needs. "They didn't just want to talk about their diets. They also tell me if they've had a stressful week; they promise to do better," she says. But Vivian is careful never to be judgmental—even when someone has a gainer week. "I ask them what they wish they had done differently. Then I'd challenge them to put it behind them. That was last week! Now let's make healthy lifestyle choices for this week." And, of course, Vivian helps them focus on God, rather than the stress or unhappiness of the previous week. "We pray to have a healthier body, not just for self-gratification, but for God."

Vivian and her team keep the records to update our database each week—her logs help track individual and team weight loss by pounds, by percentage and by BMI. She comments, "When I teach other community nutrition classes, I have never seen the success of any program like I see in this program. I think what we see here will last for a long time because they are doing it for God—for the right reason."

Another option to having live speakers is to use the videos in the Bod4God Media Kit. These videos are designed to be a perfect complement to this book (available at www.bod4god.org). The goal is to provide information to motivate and equip competitors to move forward with their healthy lifestyle choices.

Team Time

But the big-group sessions are just the beginning. Most competitors really connect with the program when they break into their small group teams. They begin by naming themselves a fruit or vegetable. In their small group they go over the information in this book and specifically discuss the weekly Victory Guide assignments.

This is a nonthreatening time to interact with the material, to share ideas on what works and what doesn't work for each person. We cheer for successes. We encourage where needed and, most of all, we pray with each other. The teams build relationships so strong that they pray for each other all week long. Some call or email each other to keep lines of communication open between the Sunday meetings.

As our first competition wound down, I heard more than a few competitors wish aloud that they could keep meeting with their teams over the summer because they attributed their weight-loss success and much of their spiritual growth to their team relationships. For most participants, the team time is the highlight of the program.

Exercise Time

In addition to the Sunday evening sessions, our church opens its doors to competitors and events even for those not signed up for the competition. The Body & Soul team, led by Dr. Liz Berbano, offers group exercise four times a week with weekday, evening and weekend options. She loves this program because each session contains elements of spiritual and physical exercise. The "cardio and strength training to contemporary Christian music," program provide an inspirational, safe, modest setting where people of all ages and abilities can work out together in a nonthreatening environment—while filling their minds with biblical messages.

Victory Celebration

The competition concludes with a Victory celebration. It is a very exciting event. The joyous emotion in the room is incredible. The individual teams first gather together to discuss the content of week 12 in this book. After this special time, all the teams gather together to celebrate their overall weight-loss results and to announce our biggest losing team and individual loser.

A Big Finish!

With such a winning program going on for so many weeks, we wanted to plan a big finale for our first competition—one that would top our opening luncheon and yet be consistent with all the Bod4God progress we'd all made. We planned a 5K run/walk. We advertised and opened it up to the community. It was a program wrap-up, a celebration and a community outreach—all rolled into one.

The 5K path started and ended on our church property, and we were able to get professional runners to help establish the route. We walked the route several Sunday evenings before the event, and we enlisted volunteers from the congregation to help along the route on race day. We found a number of corporate sponsors to donate prizes and products for the event, and after a few planning meetings, we were ready to run the race.

Finally, when race day came, 350 people participated, many of whom were among the 150 Losing to Live competitors, and many more who were from the community at large. It was an event deemed a success by all.

Competitor Damon Johnson said, "My wife, Charlene, and I enjoyed the fellowship, running for Jesus against obesity and the healthy brunch you provided for all of us. Keep on encouraging all God's people to be the best that God wants them to be and inspiring them all to enjoy eating healthy, exercising and staying faithful to the Lord by doing His will."

The Losing to Live 5K run/walk is now an annual event at our church.

A Model for a Team Competition

I want to share with you some details for how you can do a team competition in your church or organization.

How to Get Started

Starting a Losing to Live competition ministry can be a very rewarding experience! Everywhere you look these days—on the television, in books and newspaper articles—a main topic of conversation seems to be on health and weight loss. If you have a burden to address the issue of good health and weight loss with those you come in contact with, especially in your local church or another organization, then why not start a Losing to Live team competition ministry.

So you might ask, "How do I get started?" First commit the matter to prayer. Be sure to follow God's lead and not your own. Also ask around to see if there are people interested in such a program.

The next step is to meet with your pastor or appointed leader. Communicate the need for the program in your local church. When your pastor is out in the community, he probably notices that there are a lot of people who are overweight. He certainly sees people in his own congregation who suffer from obesity. This really is a *growing* problem and needs to be addressed not just by the media outlets but by the churches. Make sure your pastor is aware that Christians are the most overweight people group in America.

Share with the pastor the fact that Losing to Live was developed through much Bible study and prayer by Pastor Steve Reynolds, who weighed over 340 pounds and was diagnosed with diabetes. Through following biblical principles, Pastor Reynolds lost more than 100 pounds and is no longer diabetic. Explain that Losing to Live will show people how to lose weight and keep it off through establishing a Bod4God lifestyle. Highlight the four keys to this program, which are:

1. **D**edication: Honoring God with Your Body
2. **I**nspiration: Motivating Yourself for Change
3. **E**at and Exercise: Managing Your Habits
4. **T**eam: Building Your Circle of Support

Next, communicate the benefits of the program. The program is biblically based, which means that participants will be spending more time in God's Word. It's an opportunity for church members to work as a team to achieve good health. Also, people who may otherwise speak only in passing will have a chance to build relationships through time spent together in a group setting.

Another great benefit of the program is its appeal to people outside the church. What an opportunity for outreach. So many people have tried all the other diet plans and failed. For those people, a God-centered plan would be a new approach to an age-old problem. Also, there are people with questions about God that have no desire to attend church but would become involved in a weight-loss program. The exposure to godly principles could spark a desire to learn more about God. This could eventually lead to an increase in church participation from the surrounding community.

You must consider the space you'll need and its availability. You will need adequate space at the church, or wherever you meet. You'll need to discuss what days and the times you can meet. Share that participants will meet once a week for 12 weeks and that each session will last for 90 minutes. You will need a space for all the participants to meet together for the first 30 minutes, a place for the individual teams to meet together for the final 60 minutes, and a private place to put your scale for the weigh-in. You will also need to know what's required to properly maintain and care for the facility. Will you have childcare available and, if so, what will be the cost? If you need financial assistance to get started, explain that the funds for the materials will be recovered from the participants.

Then ask your pastor to endorse the program from the pulpit and possibly through personal participation. Most people will follow their leader. If the Pastor doesn't want to be involved, ask if he will allow you to develop a Losing to Live team challenge in the church and recruit others who may be interested.

Allow your pastor time to consider this ministry and pray about it, and then follow up. If the pastor says no, then respect that decision. If the pastor says yes, then make it happen. Follow the step-by-step guide for a successful group competition in Appendix D (pages 249-253).

What It Takes to Lead a Group of "Losers"

In Luke 6:39-40, Jesus says, "Can the blind lead the blind? Will they not both fall into the ditch? A disciple is not above his teacher, but everyone who is perfectly trained will be like his teacher." Here are some tips to help you be a good leader.

Key Information for Key Leaders

Here is some key information for those who will be leading a team of "losers":

- Remember that the No. 1 Law of Leadership is that everything rises and falls on the quality of the leadership. If you have volunteered to lead a team, spend some time in prayer about the responsibility you have taken on. How can you make your leadership sparkle and light the way for the participants on your team?

- Success in our program is measured primarily by weight loss.

- Losing to Live exists to teach people how to lose weight and keep if off through a Bod4God lifestyle. This includes four keys to a better body: (1) Dedication: honoring God with my body; (2) Inspiration: motivating myself to change; (3) Eat and exercise: learning to manage my habits; (4) team: building a circle of support whether I am losing on my own or with a team.

Team Captain Responsibilities

Here are four ways to help your team lose if you are chosen as a team captain:

1. Lead your team by example, modeling the four keys to a better body
2. Oversee your team by following the best practices
3. Study and prayerfully prepare for your team meetings
4. Encourage your team through regular communications

Meeting Schedule

Weekly team meetings at our church are held on Sunday night from 6:00 to 7:30 P.M. The format for these meetings is as follows:

- 6:00 to 6:30 P.M. We meet as one group for information and sit together as teams. We announce our overall total competition and weekly weight loss and our top competition and weekly losing team and individual loser. We have an expert speak on a health topic, especially as it relates to weight loss.

- 6:30 to 7:30 P.M. We meet for inspiration as individual teams in classrooms. The focus during this time is going over the material in this book, particularly the weekly Victory Guide assignment.

Weigh-in Procedure

Weigh-ins are done each Saturday from 9:00-11:00 A.M. and each Sunday from 9:15 to 10:00 A.M. and from 4:45 to 5:50 P.M. and from 7:30 to 8:00 P.M. Every competitor is asked to weigh in at least eight times during the competition. We ensure that each competitor has privacy during his or her weigh-in.

Each week the team captains are emailed a report showing the individual and team results from the weigh-in. In addition, each week during our opening time in the auditorium we will report on the top three team losers and top individual loser. This helps maintain overall motivation and team encouragement, both as a team and as individuals.

The weight-loss competition is based on the *percentage* of weight loss, not the *amount* of weight loss.

Weekly Assignments

Participants go through this book a week at a time. Many competitors like to go through the book twice before moving on to our alumni program. Alumni students go through a First Place 4 Health study. Individual team discussions focus on the Victory Guide assignments.

Group Rules

There are two basic group rules. First, the confidentiality rule: What is shared in the group stays in the group (unless permission is given to share the information outside of the group). Second, the conversation rule: You can only participate in the group discussion if you did the weekly assignment. Otherwise, you must just listen to others.

What to Do Next

Once you complete Bod4God, your goal should be to establish an ongoing wellness ministry. New people should go through Bod4God, and I reccommend First Place 4 Health as a follow-up. First Place 4 Health is a faith-based weight loss plan supported and endorsed by registered dietitians and physicians. Meeting in weekly support groups, the members follow a 12-week curriculum that is centered around achieving balance in four essential areas of their lives: emotional, spiritual, mental and physical. Through the program, First Place 4 Health members learn how to be victorious over past eating patterns and how to commit their minds and, ultimately, their bodies to God.

The First Place 4 Health program has delivered faith-based health and weight management instruction and support to small groups meeting in churches since 1981. It has been active in more than 12,000 churches, with more than a half million successful members! The program points members to God's strength and creates a compassionate support group that helps members stay accountable in a positive environment.

The following success story from Kevin and Tamara Fisher, a couple who practiced the First Place 4 Health program, portrays the healthy lifestyles that result from the practical disciplines of the program:

Tamara and I have been immensely blessed in losing 250 pounds together by following the balanced, Christ-centered program of First Place 4 Health. The blessings have continued far beyond weight loss. All areas of our life have been impacted, from the physical to the spiritual. In addition, our marriage, family and friends have been inspired and changed.

While our relationship has always been a blessing, it is stronger than ever before. As we moved closer to Christ as individuals, we found that our marriage was benefiting too. Our desires had aligned and our motivations changed in a profound way as we each sought to make Christ first in our lives. Gaining health enables us to share new experiences together as we train and race in triathlons, adventure races and running events. Crossing the finish line is an amazing experience, but crossing the finish line with your spouse is an even greater experience. As "Mom" and "Dad," we are better equipped to teach our four children many valuable lessons.

Today, our family leads an active, healthy and spiritual lifestyle. We talk about the foods we eat, the decisions we make and the long-term impact they can have on your body. We encourage quiet time, biblical learning and fellowship with friends and family. We enjoy television and video games, but we also enjoy soccer and cycling. In addition to an active

Before

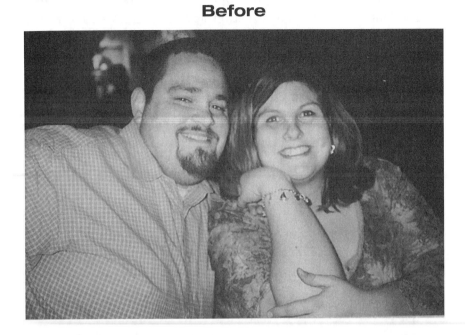

After

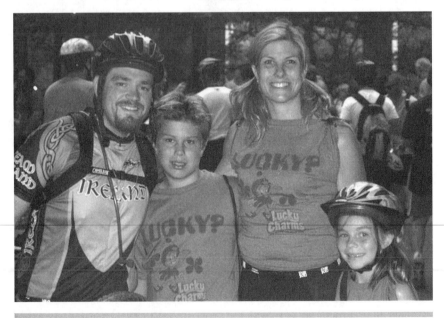

lifestyle, our two oldest children recently joined us in a 20-mile urban adventure race. Such an accomplishment was a confidence boost for the entire family, and we have plans to compete in additional races in the future. God's role in our life is evident to those around us, and we are eager to share His story.

Many of our friends have been inspired to join First Place 4 Health and now have great testimonies themselves. In addition, Tamara's mother and sisters have also joined with great results. Tamara's sister, Alexi, started First Place 4 Health wearing a size 16 and now wears a size 6. Marvin, my brother, lost approximately 60 pounds through the First Place 4 Health lifestyle. Our family has been forever changed as we strive to place Christ first in our lives.

Start a Losing to Live Weight Loss Competition

Ecclesiastes 4:9-12, the Bible tells us that teamwork produces: (1) mutual success, (2) mutual support, and (3) mutual strength. Your participation in the "Losing to Live" weight-loss competition will allow you to experience the power of teamwork as related to your health and weight loss.

Teamwork through a "Losing to Live" competition produces tremendous results. We do three competitions a year in our church and have now lost more than 12,000 pounds—that is over six tons of weight loss. Other churches and organizations are doing this competition and are seeing tremendous results.

I urge you to start this program in your church or organization and help me change lives one pound at a time.

For more information or to get a complete Bod4God Media Kit, which includes videos and other group starter tools (such as forms and promotional helps), please visit www.bod4god.org or contact me at the following:

Losing to Live
P.O Box 300, Merrifield, VA 22116
703-635-7100 · 866-596-6008

A Bod4God Close-Up

Patricia Dutchie
Lost 21 pounds

Before   **After**

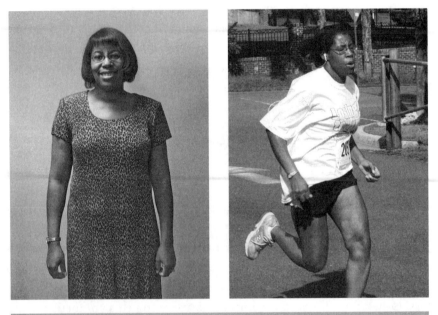

I was one of the first Bod4God team leaders, and I have been a leader three times. Our teams take on vegetable names, so my three teams were: Rutabagas, Sweet Potatoes and Beets.

Weight maintenance is difficult, but being a team leader helps you maintain your weight loss.

A team leader is a cheerleader for his or her team. "Roota-roota-roota-baga!" my first team chanted every Sunday night. We definitely had the loudest group, and we boasted three of the top 10 losers. In 20 weeks, my team lost a combined total of 297 pounds. In the second competition, my team had both the highest percentage of weight and the most weight lost.

Part of the success of a team like this comes from keeping up the enthusiasm of the team members. You must lead by example. Encouragement is so important. I learned while attending West Point that you must keep your people informed. I try to do that for my team. I send my team members motivational emails and give them prayer support. Our prayer list is long, and each member's concerns receive special attention from teammates.

One team member and one of our biggest losers, Diane Cornell, credits Bible study, accountability and my constant cajoling as contributing to her weight loss. Diane shared with our team that when her granddaughters were with her, they would say, "Grandma, did you learn your verses?" then grandmother and granddaughters would learn them together. Reports like that thrill my heart.

When we gain weight, the weight gain is not the issue. Some of the people in a couple of my groups had experienced rape; many of them felt ugly; others had suffered through other childhood trauma. There is always a root issue that causes people to gain weight. I facilitate open and honest conversation that, of course, must be kept confidential.

Ultimately, it is the Word of God that will help you lose weight. It is foundational to weight loss. The Victory Guide has a place where there is a chart of verses and a place to write a snapshot of what each verse means to you. I encourage team members to do that exercise.

In order for a person to thrive in the group, he or she must feel safe. I often remind members that a cord of three strands is not easily broken (see Eccles. 4:12.) They don't have to lose weight alone. The team will be there to help them through the tough places. And it works for them just as it worked for me.

Small Steps to Life Ideas

We are approaching the end of this book and of our 12-week Losing to Live competition. Hopefully, you have lost weight and have become healthier and stronger. Here are a few last small steps for continuing toward your goal.

What Do You Need to Know About H_2O?

Water. Once more, don't forget it. One participant drinks 40 ounces of water before 9:00 A.M. That way, the bulk of her water intake is finished early in the day.

Small Food Steps

No eating after 6 P.M. except water-based fruits. When you hit a plateau, go to an all-vegetarian lifestyle to shift to the next weight goal. Eat a lot of "living food" (raw or unprocessed) and limit eating "dead food" (chemically processed or without nutrients). Living food is made by God; it is nutritious and leads to health and life. Dead food is made by man, it is toxic and leads to illness and death.

Living Food	Dead Food
God	Man
Nutritious	Toxic
Wellness	Illness
Life	Death

If you want to live, you have to eat a lot of living food!

Small Exercise Steps

Walk 30 minutes at lunchtime on a treadmill. Or better, get out in the sunshine to walk. Walk in place or do simple exercises while waiting for something in your home: water to boil, microwave to beep, during the news and so on. And stop using power tools outside and go manual—snow shoveling, grass cutting, raking leaves, sweeping the sidewalks rather than using a blower all burn calories.

Small Steps to Life Record

What "Skinny Things" Will You Do This Week?

Fill out this chart each week by indicating: (1) What you will do to eat less to live; (2) What you will do to exercise more to live; and (3) What average daily ounces of water you will drink. Pick only a few things, and stick with them. Remember that weight loss and maintenance requires you to *eat less* and *exercise more*.

Sun.	
Mon.	
Tues.	
Wed.	
Thurs.	
Fri.	
Sat.	

Bod4God Victory Guide

To apply the information in this chapter to your life, work through the Victory Guide. It will equip you to practice the four keys to weight loss. Big losers make the Victory Guide a high priority. Record this week's weight change on "My Progress Report" located in appendix A.

Week Ten: *T* Is for Team: A Group Competition

Memory Verse
"Two are better than one, because they have a good reward for their labor" (Eccles. 4:9).

Reflection/Application Questions
1. Read Ecclesiastes 4:9. What is the value of having a team?

    _____

    _____

    _____

    _____

    _____

    _____

2. Think of a time when you had to face a struggle on your own, and then compare this to a time when you had a team to help you through a struggle. How was the team helpful to you, and how does this apply to your overall struggle to become healthy?

    _____

    _____

    _____

    _____

    _____

    _____

3. Read Hebrews 10:24-25 and Ecclesiastes 4:9-12. According to these verses, what is the value of a team?

_____

_____

_____

_____

_____

_____

_____

_____

4. In what lasting ways has God used the Losing to Live weight-loss challenge to motivate you in becoming a loser?

_____

_____

_____

_____

_____

_____

_____

_____

5. Having a lifestyle plan will greatly benefit your health. What changes do you still need to make in the following areas in order to bring about lasting results in your life?

Dedication: Honoring God with my body

_____

_____

_____

_____

_____

_____

Inspiration: Motivating myself for change

_____

_____

_____

_____

_____

_____

Eat and Exercise: Managing my habits

_____

_____

_____

_____

_____

_____

Team: Building my circle of support

_____

_____

_____

_____

_____

6. On a scale of 1 to 10, how would you evaluate your health improvements and weight loss since starting this competition? In what ways have you seen your health improve?

_____

_____

_____

_____

_____

My Bod4God Journal

Teach me, O Lord, the way of Your statutes, and I shall keep it to the end.
PSALM 119:33

Record what God is telling you to do this week to apply the four keys to a better body.

Dedication: Honoring God with My Body

_____
_____
_____
_____
_____

Inspiration: Motivating Myself for Change

_____
_____
_____
_____
_____

Eat and Exercise: Managing My Habits

_____
_____
_____
_____

Team: Building My Circle of Support

_____
_____
_____
_____

Frequently Asked Questions

*But sanctify the Lord God in your hearts, and always be ready
to give a defense to everyone who asks you a reason for the
hope that is in you, with meekness and fear.*

1 PETER 3:15

QUESTION 1
What are your four keys to a better body?

People ask me, "How did you lose weight?" I tell them, "There are four
keys to weight loss." They are:

1. *Dedication:* For me, weight loss was a matter of bringing together my belief system and my behavior. I knew what the
   Bible taught, yet my behavior didn't reflect it. Bringing belief and behavior together meant dedicating my body to
   God and honoring Him with my body. My biggest breakthrough was realizing that I needed to depend on God to
   help me. I couldn't do it alone. There's plenty of evidence
   to demonstrate that some people can lose weight and get
   healthy without God, but I'm not one of them. I needed
   God to help me. I had to learn to incorporate walking in
   the Spirit, not just in the pulpit, but also in improving my
   health. I had to bring those two together in my life.

2. *Inspiration.* To get started and stay on track, you have to find out what motivates you. The fact that you are reading this book is a good start. John 10:10 is the key verse for me in that area. Jesus said, "The thief does not come except to steal, and to kill, and to destroy. I have come that they may have life, and that they may have it more abundantly." The thief, Satan, has an agenda for your life and mine. He comes to steal, kill and destroy. For many of us, he is using a knife and a fork to do it. Many times, we want to lose weight for some special event. Maybe there's a high school reunion coming up, or a wedding or some big family event for which you'd like to lose weight. Maybe you do lose weight, but when that event is over, what happens then? Do you gain the weight back? Probably. That's because poor eating habits and lack of movement have become a way of life for you and you still haven't changed your lifestyle. My inspiration is that I want to live the abundant life Jesus promised, and I want it in both quality and in quantity.

3. *Eat and Exercise.* I knew I had to manage my habits. I had to learn 1 Thessalonians 4:4, "Each of you should know how to possess his own vessel." "Vessel" here means "body." I had to learn how to possess my body better by improving my habits of eating and exercising—essentially, eating less and exercising more.

4. *Team.* I needed other people to help me in my journey. Proverbs 27:17 says, "As iron sharpens iron, so a man sharpens the countenance of his friend." I had to bring people into my life who could sharpen me when it came to moving toward better health. I had to bring into my life people who knew things I needed to know about health. I had to allow them to impact my life through books, one-on-one encounters, and group-type settings.

QUESTION 2
Can I apply these keys to other addictions in my life?

Yes. These are transferable concepts. In other words, these keys can apply to other areas of your life in which you struggle.

The Losing to Live message started with a sermon series that took the principle of "losing weight to live better and longer" and showed the ways in which it applies to lots of different areas. We talked about problem areas that have their basis on elevating self above God's Word:

- *Debt* is usually all about self—buying things you can't afford, and getting yourself in debt.

- *Anger* is about self. "You offended me. I'm angry with you, and I have a right to be angry."

- *Lust* is about looking at what you want to look at. It's about a strong desire to do what you want to do. It's about acting the way you want to act.

- *Stress* has its roots in an attitude that says, "I can get through life all by myself. I don't need God or anyone else to help me." The same principles apply. In Galatians 2:20, Paul said, "I have been crucified with Christ; it is no longer I who live, but Christ lives in me." It's about dying to self and letting Christ live in and through you.

These principles can be transferred to other areas of your life. As an example, let's use the acrostic D.I.E.T. in dealing with financial debt.

- *Dedication.* Just start out saying, "God, my money belongs to You. You are the owner of it. I'm going to honor You with my money."

- *Inspiration.* Be inspired by reading books about how others have overcome their debt—particularly credit card debt. Mary Hunt's book *Debt-Proof Your Marriage: How to Achieve Financial Harmony* tells you how not to accumulate stress-inducing debt; or Dave Ramsey's books on financial freedom are available at all bookstores. Both Mary and Dave had huge debt and had to figure out a way to overcome it. They can inspire you.

- *Eat and exercise.* Managing your Habits. Maybe you have a bad habit of loading up your credit cards with debt. Cut them up. Maybe you have always bought the best of everything—food, clothing, cars. Take another look at your habits and see if you really need top of the line products to accomplish your goals.

- *Team.* Team up with others for whatever problems, stresses and habits are controlling your life so that you can gain control of them. Form a financial club or an investment club. Work with a team of financial people to learn how to achieve your goals.

QUESTION 3
What does the Bible mean when it says "your body is the temple of the Holy Spirit" (1 Corinthians 6:19)?

First, it means that God's Spirit is a resident in your life. The Scripture assumes that the moment you come to Christ—the moment you were saved—the Holy Spirit came into your life. Jesus said, "I will pray the Father, and He will give you another Helper, that He may abide with you forever—the Spirit of truth, whom the world cannot receive, because it neither sees Him nor knows Him; but you know Him, for He dwells with you and will be in you" (John 14:16-17). God lives in you. Think about it; you as a Christian actually house deity. God doesn't live in a church building. There is nothing sacred about a church building except that it is a place where we come together to corporately worship the Lord. Our bodies are sacred because they are God's temples.

Second, it means that we are to reflect the glory of God. In 1 Corinthians 6:20, Paul says, "For you were bought with a price, therefore glorify God in your body." Because my body is His temple, I should treat it accordingly. In 1 Corinthians 10:31, Paul says, "Therefore, whether you eat or drink or whatever you do, do all to the glory of God."

The Bible tells us that one of the ways we can glorify God is through what we eat and what we drink.

QUESTION 4
Does Jesus care whether a person is skinny or fat?

That's an interesting question. I'm not questioning whether Jesus loves us—of course He does. At the same time, He also wants us to be healthy, and that includes not being overweight. He is all about us living. The Bible says He gave His precious blood so that we could live (see John 6:33-35; 1 John 5:11-12).

I have never doubted the love of God in my life. He doesn't love me any more today because I lost weight. But He does care, and He's delighted that I've lost weight. He knows I can live better and probably longer because of my weight loss.

Jesus was nailed to the cross. He suffered and died there because He wanted us to live for all eternity with Him. He also wants us to enjoy our journey here on earth. He cares about our weight problems. He came to give us eternal life in heaven and abundant life on this earth. Being at a proper weight and staying active will give us a better and more abundant life here on earth. So remember that God is not going to love you any less or any more because you lose weight or don't lose weight. It's not about His love, but He does care.

QUESTION 5
Is overeating a sin?

Yes, it is a sin! In 1 Thessalonians 5:23, Paul writes, "Now may the God of peace Himself sanctify you completely; and may your whole spirit, soul, and body be preserved blameless at the coming of our Lord Jesus Christ." God wants to sanctify us wholly—that means our whole spirit and body. Part of being sanctified is having a sanctified eating pattern. So, yes, I think the Bible bears out God's perspective that overeating is a sin.

QUESTION 6
What is your eating and exercise plan?

This is a popular question because people always want to know how I lost weight and how I am keeping it off. There are many ways to lose weight. I've had lots of people try to get me to adopt various plans. They say, "We've got to come see you, and you've got to tell everybody about our plan." That plan may be wonderful. It probably will work for some people, but I'm not about endorsing a single plan. I believe you can lose weight lots of different ways.

The problem isn't that we don't have enough plans. The problem is that we don't stick to the plans or haven't found the right plan for us. My wife and I are not on the same plan. She is losing weight, but she's not losing it the way I am. We are cool with that. She's excited about what she's doing. It's working for her, and I'm proud of her.

What's working for me is a kind of low-carb plan—I guess. I'm eating some carbs but not loading up on them. What I eat is too boring for most people. I'm a boring guy. I don't have to have a lot of variety of foods in my life to be happy—at least not in this season of life.

A lot of you are different in that way. You've got to come up with all kinds of fresh ideas. You get your cookbooks out and make this and cook that. I'm not that way. Here's what I've begun doing pretty much every day since I embarked on my weight-loss journey:

- *Breakfast:* I start my day by eating a nutritional bar. My favorite is the CLIF® bar. It's very nutritious, and I like it a lot. I'll eat one or sometimes two a day. I eat an apple, sometimes two a day. With breakfast I drink 32 ounces of water, and yes, I also drink coffee. On my day off, I'll sometimes fix eggs for breakfast. On Wednesday, we have our staff meeting, and somebody fixes us eggs. I will typically eat those.

- *Lunch:* For lunch I get a grilled chicken salad with lowfat dressing. I drink more water. If I go out to eat, that's what I order. A lot of times, I'll just go to a fast-food place or grocery store and pick up different salads. Most fast-food places have a lowfat grilled chicken salad of some kind. On my day off, I'll make my own salad.

- *Dinner:* For dinner I have lean meat; and five out of seven days a week, that lean meat is chicken. I have green vegetables like broccoli or green beans, and diet soda. Then I have some fruit, like an orange or grapes. Many times I'll also have some low-fat yogurt.

- *Snacks:* Planned snacks are important to losing weight. Snacking properly can help keep your metabolism functioning at its peak. I have a late afternoon snack or an early evening snack. This could be a second CLIF bar, a piece of fruit or a few almonds.

Friday night is my "cheat night," but the longer I am on the program, the less I need to cheat. In the beginning it was the most wonderful day in the world. I funneled all my cravings into cheat night. If I had been craving ice cream all week, I'd think, *Just two more days until I can go get my ice cream.* But the longer I go on with my small steps to life, the less I need this fix.

I'm on a lifestyle plan, and what that means is that if there is a very special event (I don't try to find a special event every day) like Christmas, I will eat my Christmas meal. I have a good time at the event. I plan to do this the rest of my life. On my plan, you eat Christmas dinner and you enjoy it without guilt. I do try to watch my portion size at the special event. Also, if I know I will be eating a lot at one meal, I cut back at other meals.

Regarding my exercise plan, I started out very slowly. The biggest mistake people make in exercise is to overdo it when they first begin. I am slowly building up my routine. Today, I go to a gym and do 35 minutes on the treadmill and 15 different weightlifting activities three times a week. I also play basketball once a week. On Sunday nights, I walk the 5K route. It works for me. I didn't learn this from a book. I didn't get it from some other person's plan. I just started doing it, and I started liking it. So I kept on doing it, and I kept on losing weight.

Again, you don't have to do what I do. I'm just offering my plan as an idea to get you going. You have to find your own plan.

QUESTION 7
How should I respond when tempted to do unhealthy things?

One of the biggest things to keep you from giving in to temptation is disciplining your mind. What you allow yourself to think about is what you do, and what you do is what you feel. If you want to change your feelings, change your doing. If you want to change your doing, change your thinking.

Every time I gave into a food temptation, my giving in started with an idea in my mind. I said, "Nice, very nice." And then I ate it. And then I felt bad. So if you want to feel better, you've got to do better. If I'm going to do better, I've got to think better. I have to change my thinking. When I think of that big Hershey's chocolate bar with almonds, I've got to cast down that imagination. I've got to bring every thought into the obedience of Christ (see 2 Cor. 10:5).

One of the Scripture verses that has helped me a lot is Galatians 6:7-8, "Do not be deceived, God is not mocked; for whatever a man sows, that he will also reap. For he who sows to his flesh will of the flesh reap corruption, but he who sows to the Spirit will of the Spirit reap everlasting life." Do you want corruption or life? I want life. So I think a lot about life, and that begins to change my feelings and my actions.

QUESTION 8
What can I do about overeating because of the stress in my life?

A lot of people eat for comfort. They're under a lot stress, so they eat. I've told you earlier, a lot of us who come from the South associate high-fat, rich foods with comfort. It's what we grew up with. It's comforting to us to eat those things.

The Bible calls us to turn to Christ rather than food. Philippians 4:6-7 says, "Be anxious for nothing, but in everything by prayer and supplication, with thanksgiving, let your requests be made known to God; and the peace of God, which surpasses all understanding, will guard your hearts and minds through Christ Jesus." There is a direct correlation between prayer and peace. And that's "peace," not "piece." Make sure you get the spelling right. What can you do about overeating because of the stress in your life? Turn to Christ rather than food.

QUESTION 9
Why does the Bible say that bodily exercise profits little?

First Timothy 4:8 is an interesting verse. We've talked about it before, but I want to highlight it here in a special way. At the time Paul wrote this verse, people had bodily exercise every day. They lived a life that was more intense physically than any gym workout today. As a carpenter, Jesus was a physical worker. In His time, people walked everywhere they went. They had no power tools or electronic conveniences to do the heavy work. Life itself was a workout. When this Scripture verse was read by its original recipients, they would have recognized immediately that it was meant to be a comparison between the physical and the spiritual.

The physical is temporary, so exercise profits the physical body a little. Spiritual exercise lasts forever. It is eternal. We need both physical and spiritual exercise. Growing Christians know that their spiritual exercise is of more eternal value than their physical exercise, yet they need physical exercise to keep the body functioning at peak efficiency.

QUESTION 10
Is it necessary to measure my food?

Men's Health magazine had a small article on writing down what you eat. It said that, "Those who kept a food record for three weeks or longer lost 3.5 pounds more than those who didn't."[1] While most men and many women don't like to write down everything they put in their mouths, (I don't write anything down, but I am very mindful about what I eat), keeping a food record appears to work. Even if you only do it for a few weeks, writing down what you eat will help you know how many calories you are actually taking in. Don't forget to write down all those bites you take while cooking or cleaning up after dinner. They all count and add up quickly.

Question 11
How can I know what I'm putting in my mouth?

Bookstores carry many varieties of calorie counter books and booklets that contain all the nutrient information you need. Many of these books are small enough to carry in your pocket so that you can consult them and make wise choices whenever you're eating at a chain restaurant or fast-food franchise. Also, most major food franchises offer their food's nutrition information online. Here's an interesting comparison of the higher-calorie-level burgers out there. I hate to even contemplate the fat grams in some of these burgers listed![2]

Example: Hamburgers	Calories
McDonald's Hamburger®	.250
Burger King's Triple Whopper with Cheese®	.1,230
McDonald's Angus Steak Burger®	.640
Jack-in-the-Box's Ultimate Cheeseburger®	.1,010
Dairy Queen's Original Burger®	.350
Dairy Queen's ¼ lb FlameThrower GrillBurger®	.840
TGI Friday's Cheesy Bacon Cheeseburger®	.1,540
Wendy's Baconator®	.840
Wendy's Triple Everything and Cheese®	.980

Notes
1. Maria Masters, ed., "Weight-Loss Bulletin: Write Off the Pounds," *Men's Health,* February 2009, p. 38.
2. This excerpt of calorie information was collected by ABC News and posted on their website at http://abcnews.go.com.

Small Steps to Life Record

What "Skinny Things" Will You Do This Week?

Fill out this chart each week by indicating: (1) What you will do to eat less to live; (2) What you will do to exercise more to live; and (3) What average daily ounces of water you will drink. Pick only a few things, and stick with them. Remember that weight loss and maintenance requires you to *eat less* and *exercise more*.

Sun.	
Mon.	
Tues.	
Wed.	
Thurs.	
Fri.	
Sat.	

Bod4God Victory Guide

To apply the information in this chapter to your life, work through the Victory Guide. It will equip you to practice the four keys to weight loss. Big losers make the Victory Guide a high priority. Record this week's weight change on "My Progress Report" located in appendix A.

Week Eleven: Frequently Asked Questions

Memory Verse

"But sanctify the Lord God in your hearts, and always be ready to give a defense to everyone who asks you a reason for the hope that is in you, with meekness and fear" (1 Pet. 3:15).

Reflection/Application Questions

Answer the following questions in your own words. How does each question apply to you? Use back-up Scripture when possible.

1. What are the four keys to a better body?

   _____

   _____

   _____

   _____

   _____

   _____

2. How can you apply these keys to other addictions in your life?

   _____

   _____

   _____

   _____

   _____

3. What does the Bible mean when it says your body is the temple of the Holy Spirit?

_____

_____

_____

_____

_____

4. Does Jesus care whether a person is skinny or fat?

_____

_____

_____

_____

_____

5. Is overeating a sin? Why or why not?

_____

_____

_____

_____

_____

6. What is your eating and exercise plan?

_____

_____

_____

_____

_____

7. How should you respond when tempted to do unhealthy things?

_____

_____

_____

_____

8. What can you do about overeating because of the stress in your life?

_____

_____

_____

_____

_____

_____

_____

9. Why does the Bible say that bodily exercise profits little?

_____

_____

_____

_____

_____

_____

_____

10. Is it necessary to measure your food? Why or why not?

_____

_____

_____

_____

_____

_____

11. How can you know what you are putting in your mouth?

_____

_____

_____

_____

_____

_____

My Bod4God Journal

Teach me, O Lord, the way of Your statutes, and I shall keep it to the end.

Psalm 119:33

Record what God is telling you to do this week to apply the four keys to a better body.

Dedication: Honoring God with My Body

_____

_____

_____

_____

_____

Inspiration: Motivating Myself for Change

_____

_____

_____

_____

_____

Eat and Exercise: Managing My Habits

_____

_____

_____

_____

Team: Building My Circle of Support

_____

_____

_____

_____

_____

Your Bod4God Lifestyle Plan

It's time to commit! Our conclusion isn't really a conclusion, it's a be-ginning—the beginning of a new way of life. So how do you get started on this new lifestyle? You do it by making a commitment.

A Scripture to guide you in your commitment is 2 Corinthians 7:1: "Therefore, having these promises, beloved, let us cleanse ourselves from all filthiness of the flesh and spirit, perfecting holiness in the fear of God."

You now have the tools you need to get on the Bod4God lifestyle path. It's time for commitment. It's time to cleanse your body from all those things that would keep you from having a Bod4God. It's time to act on what you know is true.

I've done my best to share God's Word with you. Will you make a commitment to do it? If so, fill out your Bod4God commitment form and your new Bod4God Lifestyle Plan. Sign the commitment form, and when times get tough, go back and reread the commitment you made. Follow your new lifestyle plan and continue to build on your small steps to life. You will never regret it.

My Bod4God Commitment Form

Now that you have read this book and are fully convinced you need to make lifestyle changes, it's time to make a commitment to losing weight and keeping it off.

Dedication: Honoring God with My Body

I say then: Walk in the Spirit, and you shall not fulfill the lust of the flesh.
GALATIANS 5:16

Inspiration: Motivating Myself for Change

The thief does not come except to steal, and to kill, and to destroy. I have come that they may have life, and that they may have it more abundantly.
JOHN 10:10

Eat and Exercise: Managing My Habits

Each of you should know how to possess his own vessel in sanctification and honor.
1 THESSALONIANS 4:4

Team: Building My Circle of Support

Two are better than one, because they have a good reward for their labor.
ECCLESIASTES 4:9

Knowing that my body is made by God and for God, I commit myself to a healthy lifestyle.

Name _____ Date _____

My Bod4God New Lifestyle Plan

Take time now to summarize your current lifestyle plan and the small steps to life that you have made so far. Remember, your lifestyle plan continues to be a work in progress, so keep making those small steps to life.

My New Nutritional Plan

How much water will you drink each day? (Remember: Most people should drink at least eight glasses, eight ounces each, of water per day.)

_____

_____

_____

_____

_____

_____

What will you eat for breakfast?

_____

_____

_____

_____

_____

What will you eat for lunch?

_____

_____

_____

_____

_____

What will you eat for dinner?

_____
_____
_____
_____
_____
_____
_____

What will you eat for snacks?

_____
_____
_____
_____
_____
_____

My New Exercise Plan

What kind of exercise will you do? Fill in your exercise routine in the following chart.

Sun.	
Mon.	
Tues.	
Wed.	
Thurs.	
Fri.	
Sat.	

My Progress Report

BOD 4 GOD

In order to know what progress you are making, you need a place to record where you began and whether you are losing or gaining weight. Please fill out the information requested below. Each week for 12 weeks, record your progress. It's important, so be faithful to record your progress.

Name: _Darryl Lloyd_ Start Date: _6/6/12_ End Date: _____

My Starting Weight: _251_ My Final Weight: _____

Goal: _225_

My Starting Measurements:

Neck: _____

Arm (Bicep): _____

Chest: _____

Waist: _____

Hips: _____

Thighs: _____

Calf: _____

My Ending Measurements:

Neck: _____

Arm (Bicep): _____

Chest: _____

Waist: _____

Hips: _____

Thighs: _____

Calf: _____

My Weight Loss

Week	+ / -
1	0
2	
3	
4	-3
5	-4
6	+2

Week	+ / -
7	
8	
9	
10	
11	
12	

BOD 4 GOD

Memory Verses

Then Jesus said to those Jews who believed Him, "If you abide in My word, you are My disciples indeed. And you shall know the truth, and the truth shall make you free."

JOHN 8:31-32

The Bible is the absolute truth. Jesus said that by knowing the truth we can be set free from sin. Understand that the battle of the bulge will be won or lost in the mind; therefore, fill your mind with the Word of God.

There are 11 memory verses for you to learn throughout the program. Memorize one verse each week if possible. These verses will encourage you to stay true to your goal of a better Bod4God. Write one verse on a card each week and post the card in your car, on your bathroom mirror, your computer screen or wherever you'll see it first thing in the morning.

Week One: Colossians 1:16

"For by Him all things were created that are in heaven and that are on earth, visible and invisible, whether thrones or dominions or principalities or powers. All things were created through Him and for Him."

Week Two: Matthew 16:24-25

"If anyone desires to come after Me, let him deny himself, and take up his cross, and follow Me. For whoever desires to save his life will lose it, but whoever loses his life for My sake will find it."

Week Three: Galatians 5:16

"I say then: Walk in the Spirit, and you shall not fulfill the lust of the flesh."

Week Four: Romans 10:9

"If you confess with your mouth the Lord Jesus and believe in your heart that God has raised Him from the dead, you will be saved."

Week Five: John 10:10

"The thief does not come except to steal, and to kill, and to destroy. I have come that they may have life, and that they may have it more abundantly."

Week Six: Philippians 4:13

"I can do all things through Christ who strengthens me."

Week Seven: 1 Thessalonians 4:4

"Each of you should know how to possess his own vessel in sanctification and honor."

Week Eight: 1 Corinthians 10:31

"Therefore, whether you eat or drink, or whatever you do, do all to the glory of God."

Week Nine: Psalm 51:12

"Restore to me the joy of Your salvation, and uphold me by Your generous Spirit."

Week Ten: Ecclesiastes 4:9

"Two are better than one, because they have a good reward for their labor."

Week Eleven: 1 Peter 3:15

"But sanctify the Lord God in your hearts, and always be ready to give a defense to everyone who asks you a reason for the hope that is in you, with meekness and fear."

How Other Churches Are Using the Bod4God Program

My great passion is to see this program spread to churches everywhere. And it has begun. Here is Greg Judy's inspiring story.

Greg Judy
Independent Bible Church
Martinsburg, West Virginia

I've always been heavy, and I've had 13 hip surgeries due to a degenerative disease that began between the ages of 10 and 13. I couldn't exercise at that time because of the pain in my hips, and so I sat and ate. My disease began with overweight and became worse because of my obesity.

I spent two years in and out of the hospital. They told me that by the time I was 30, I would be incapacitated. Not only my hips, but my knees were gone too. I've learned since then that being only 10 pounds overweight increases the force on the knee by 30 to 60 pounds with each step (www.hopkins-arthritis.org). That alone is reason enough to lose weight.

When I went to see the doctor at age 40, I was 300 pounds overweight. The doctor said I had to lose weight. But how could I do that? I considered bariatric surgery and went to see a doctor 70 miles from where I lived. While there, I decided that before pursuing surgery, I would try to change my eating habits. I met a guy at the clinic who was also considering bariatric surgery. I tried to talk him into trying to lose weight another way. "No," he said, "I'm going to take the easy way out." Well, he had the surgery, and three months later, he died from complications resulting from the surgery.

I began to lose weight, and when I had lost 135 pounds, I went to see Dr. Michael A. Mont at Mt. Sinai Hospital in Baltimore. He said he could now do surgery on my hips. I had the surgery and then, during 10 weeks of recovery, I put 35 pounds back on. Three years later, I had my knees replaced.

Then I heard Pastor Steve's ad on the radio. I called to check out the program and see if I could bring it to my own church in West Virginia. My wife and I had already started eating better and losing weight, but we wanted to see if the program would work at our church. We came every Sunday evening from Independent Bible Church in Martinsburg, West Virginia, an hour and a half away, to attend the sessions. I now run the program at my church. My team at home lost 446.3 pounds in our first competition. The biggest individual loser lost 32.5 pounds in 12 weeks.

I now read all kinds of healthy eating books. I look for God's principles in them. I ask, "What would Jesus eat?" Now 80 percent of my diet is fruit and vegetables. I drink a gallon of water a day and I eat six to eight meals a day. I walk faithfully on the treadmill. I started at 15 minutes a day at a flat level. Now I walk on an incline for an hour and 15 minutes a day. That's about five miles. I am thankful for Bod4God. I want to live and live well. I have four sons—17, 13, 11 and 7 years old. I want to see them grow up and I want to live to see my grandchildren. Bod4God makes that much more likely to happen.

Randy Conley
First Evangelical Lutheran Church
Floresville, Texas

Randy Conley, pastor of First Evangelical Lutheran Church in Floresville, Texas, a suburb of San Antonio, first learned of the Losing to Live competition when he saw a small article in his local newspaper copied from the Associated Press article that first appeared in the *Washington Post*. He ordered Pastor Steve's *Bod4God* book and started applying what he learned to his own life.

Pastor Conley was overweight, as were many of his parishioners. San Antonio holds the dubious title of being the third most obese city in the United States. That good old Tex-Mex food of fried tortillas, cheese, sweet tea and all kinds of fat-laden food has done its damage and packed the pounds on many of his churchgoers.

Pastor Conley had struggled alone to lose weight a few years earlier, but then, as so many do, he put it right back on. In August 2008, he set up a Losing to Live competition at his church. For his own sake, he had to get his family onboard. He had teenagers at home, and everyone knows the junk food teens can eat. He had to ask them to help him eat in a healthy way. He started eating fresh foods versus packaged foods. One of his children started eating better as an encouragement to him. She got a real bonus for her efforts. She lost two pants sizes just by changing her eating habits.

This time, using the Losing to Live competition, the weight-loss program is working for him. He weighed 286 pounds at the start of the competition, and he was rapidly climbing toward 300 pounds. He has taken off 38 pounds so far. His approach is "slow and steady." Pastor Conley attributes the intimacy of the small group as well as the scriptural basis that is emphasized in the Losing to Live competition for his success. He believes it is easier to get intimate with people who have already been there for you at other times in your life. They know you and care about you.

Thirty-five people started the competition, and 25 stuck with it. The groups' total weight loss was almost 400 pounds. One teenager lost 28 pounds. One elderly person was able to get off of prescription drugs. There were two men's groups, and Randy led those groups. Some of the men had never been in a Bible study before.

Pastor Conley believes the small group concept works because it is a safe place for people to share their struggles and successes with weight. He says that it's embarrassing to be overweight, and in the small group, people can be open about their weight issues and encourage each other. Often his group members call each other throughout the week to see how others are doing.

In his community there is a man who runs an Anytime Fitness™ gym. He is allowing those on the Losing to Live program to come in and work out at a substantial discount. One group does step aerobics. Other groups gather at one of Floresville's lovely parks to walk together.

Pastor Conley says, to other pastors who see obesity as a problem in their congregations, "Be the example. People look to their pastor for integrity, and there is so little of that around today. You can encourage others and woo them toward a better lifestyle." He says that over a period of time at church functions, the donuts have decreased and the fruit has increased. He's also noticed people are taking smaller portions of food at those events. Losing to Live is working in this Texas church.

Cathy Bowser
First United Church of Christ
Pittsburgh, Pennsylvania

Cathy Bowser of Pittsburgh, Pennsylvania, had been involved in many different types of weight-loss programs. She would lose weight and after awhile regain it. Her weight had yo-yoed over the years. Then her health was in jeopardy. "I was ruining my health," she says. "I knew God had created me and I had a purpose in life." She didn't know what to do except ask God to help her. One day, when she was looking for books on the Amazon website, she saw Pastor Steve's first book on weight loss as one of the "suggested books." She ordered the book, read it and decided not only to try the plan herself but also get together a group at her church so they could support one another.

That's how the First United Church of Christ began its Losing to Live competition. There were 10 people who attended the competition for a total loss of 168 lbs. For the exercise part of the competition, she devised a program she calls "Let's Move." Because there are several people in the group who have health issues and can't really do strenuous aerobics, they are using DVDs that have sitting exercises.

Cathy thinks this plan works where others have failed because of the support that participants receive from each other. Everyone has a partner. All the members of the group have each other's telephone numbers, and she encourages them to call each other during the week. The partners weigh each other and keep the weight private between them but record it as a "loss-in" instead of a "weigh-in." She says, "This keeps everything positive." For example, she chooses a positive theme for each week. "A theme will come out of the blue," she says. "One of them was, 'The Lord is my portion.'" Another positive way to approach weight loss is not to call exercise "exercise." She calls it "movement."

She says their church is small but their pastor is very progressive. He is totally supportive of the effort she is making to help God's people have healthier bodies. He believes God gives people spiritual gifts, and when they have an idea or a passion to do something, he tells them to run with it. So Cathy ran with her passion. She says, "God is honored in even the small things you attempt; so do the small things."

Barbara Coghlan
Grace Community Chapel
St. Peters, Missouri (a suburb of St. Louis)

Barbara Coghlan, outreach director for her church, learned about Bod4God when a lady from her church heard about the program on the *700 Club*. "She asked if I would be interested in pursuing having a Losing to Live competition. I said yes." First Barbara ran a test group to see if the program worked and as a place where she could train leaders. Twelve people finished that competition, and they finished strong. They lost more than 200 pounds as a group. Barbara has lost 50 pounds so far.

"From that first group we expanded to our church and community," she says. "This time, in our second competition, we had 50 in the group, and our weight loss was 636 lbs. There were 11 men in this competition. Losing to Live works for men. "I think it works for men because this is not a diet. It is, rather, a way to honor God with our lives," Barbara said.

"It's true that meeting with a group provides accountability, but it's more than just meeting with a group. The choices we are making for God make the big difference. When looking at the problem of overweight, this plan is not about dieting but about how we can honor God with our eating."

Making small steps to life, rather than dieting, and memorizing Scripture is powerful. Barbara says that the Scripture, "Walk in the Spirit, and you will not fulfill the lust of the flesh" (Gal. 5:16), got to her heart. It caused her to look at Scripture in a new way and begin applying Scripture to her eating. It was the whole concept of walking in the Spirit and recognizing that it was God who created us.

"Our pastor is supportive and excited about the program. He doe not need to lose weight, so he is not part of the group as a competitor, but he asks questions to see how we are doing. He sees this as a huge opportunity for our church in terms of outreach."

Barbara wanted a biblically based program for weight loss, and this was the right one for her and her church. It has just the right blend of support, encouragement and the Word of God. Barbara acknowledges that when she began the first competition she was in a terrible mood. She was sure she would fail as she had so many times. But she has been successful at losing weight. She knows that going forward and maintaining her weight loss will be difficult, but she believes that the lifestyle changes she has made will help her maintain her weight.

Glenn Clary
Anchorage Baptist Temple
Anchorage, Alaska

Dr. Jerry Prevo is the pastor of one of Alaska's largest and most influential churches. He first learned about Bod4God from a magazine article. Dr. Prevo asked Pastor Steve to present the Losing to Live competition to his church and then appointed a staff member, Pastor Glenn Clary, to lead the program.

Pastor Clary said, "I first learned about the Bod4God lifestyle and book when Pastor Steve sent a letter of introduction to Dr. Prevo, and he introduced me to the program and asked me to lead a group.

"So far we have only had one competition, but it was successful. Personally, I lost 23 pounds, and the group lost 279 pounds. I think the program works because it is strong on the spiritual aspect of diet change as well as in making small incremental changes.

"I believe that Losing to Live provides participants with hope that change is possible. Many people live day after day with no hope of things ever getting better. A Losing to Live support group provides that hope. It's a hope for spiritual and physical change."

How to Set up Your Competition

Can individuals lose weight without being believers—without God? Can they lose weight without a competition? Yes, they can, but it is our experience that people do best when they first commit their weight problem to God and then ask for His help on a daily basis. They also do well when they are part of a competition in which they are encouraged by others to take those steps that will help them lose weight. I believe with all my heart that a competition is essential to weight loss. We all need connection and a place to share our successes and failures. So don't try to lose weight alone—join a team of losers!

Here is a simple guide for setting up a Losing to Live Weight Loss Competition.

What to Do Before the Competition

Step 1: Know Your Purposes

If you are clear about your purposes and can articulate them to a pastor, to key leaders and to a congregation, you will quickly gain their approval. Christians are the most overweight people group in America, and Losing to Live has been designed to confront and solve this problem. This program will show people in your church how to lose weight and keep it off through a Bod4God lifestyle. The bottom line is changing lives one pound at a time.

Step 2: Seek Approval from the Leadership of Your Church

- If you are the *pastor*, inform your key leaders what you are planning to do and why you are doing it.

- If you are *not the pastor*, go first to your pastor and share your passion to help church members to lose weight. Let the pastor inform the key leaders.

- Tell all those in leadership what the program will cost the church in terms of dollars for advertising, purchasing the participant kits (if the church is going to provide any of the kits for participants—see step 9 below), coffee, snacks or lunches and any other expenses you foresee. Tell the leadership how you plan to fund the program (e.g., through offerings, registration fees or fundraisers).

Step 3: Establish Your Location

The entire competition takes 12 weeks. Participants meet once a week for 90 minutes. During the first 30 minutes, everyone will meet together to share his or her results and hear from a speaker. During the remaining 60 minutes, participants will break into teams for discussion. Keeping this in mind, you will need:

- A place large enough for all participants to meet together such as an auditorium, multipurpose room, or fellowship hall.
- Smaller rooms where individual teams can meet.
- A private place to put your scale for weigh-ins.

Step 4: Determine Your Schedule

For an idea of how to set up your schedule, see chapter 10 for the schedule that we have used successfully at my church. Remember that the total time for a meeting is 90 minutes, which includes 30 minutes for the total group rally time and 60 minutes for the small group time.

Step 5: Recruit and Assign Leaders

You will need a director, team captains and administrative support to do the weigh-ins and other activities during the sessions. Think long and pray earnestly about who these people should be, as they will be crucial to the success of the program. Specifically, seek out those who will be able to:

- *Educate the participants.* These people may include doctors, nutritionists, physical coaches and others in your congregation with certain areas of expertise.

- *Encourage the participants through worship and devotional times.* These people may include those who have themselves lost weight and know how long and difficult the process can be.

- *Equip the participants.* Look for people who can help train the participants with regard to eating healthy and exercising. Look around, and you will be sure to find someone who is leading a Pilates or aerobics class or who is known for his or her healthy cooking. Press them into service for this program.

Step 6: Organize Your Registration Process

All participants must fill out a Losing to Live registration form (this is part of the Bod4God Media Kit and can be obtained at www.bod4god.org). Collect these well in advance of the competition. (You will need this information to properly order your participant kits.)

Step 7: Implement Your Promotion Strategy

Your promotion should target your church and community. A promotional video and other materials are available at www.bod4god.org.

Step 8: Host an Orientation Meeting

Two to three weeks before the first competition, host an orientation meeting for potential participants. The goal is to explain how it works and then register participants for the upcoming 12-week competition. Distribute the Losing to Live Fact Sheet and show the orientation video presentation by Pastor Steve Reynolds, both of which are part of the Bod4God Media Kit and are available at www.bod4god.org.

Step 9: Order Your Participant Kits

I recommend that each participant obtain an official Losing to Live Weight Loss Kit (available at www.bod4god.org), which contains the

Bod4God trade book, by Pastor Steve Reynolds (each participant will need a book to do the Victory Guide exercises and other exercises that are a crucial element to success in the program) and an official Losing to Live T-shirt.

Step 10: Determine Your Teams

After each participant has been registered, divide the enrollees into teams of 6 to 12 people. Each team should be balanced out between those who need to lose a lot of weight and those who need to lose less weight. Don't worry if you have only one or two teams the first time. As these first teams have success, others will notice and join the program.

Step 11: Set up Your Weigh-in Procedure

You will need a good-quality scale and a private place for the weigh-in—setting up the scale in a classroom is often ideal. Have participants come in one at a time to weigh in to respect their privacy. For the convenience of participants, you may want to schedule several weigh-in times.

Step 12: Set up How You Will Communicate with Participants

Get email addresses and phone numbers from all participants. For the best success, the director and the group leader need to be in contact with the participants on a weekly basis. (A few "atta boys" will encourage participants to stay on track.)

What to Do During the Competition

Step 1: Conduct Weekly Weigh-in

Record the participant's weight each week without comment. Whether they have lost of gained weight, this is their story to tell. Say nothing to the participant or anyone else.

Step 2: Conduct Weekly Rally Time

At the rally, announce individual teams' total weight loss. Individuals will also be competing to be one of the top 10 losers of the 12-week competition. Also, line up a speaker for each rally. Have an "expert" speak about exercise, nutrition or attitude. These individuals can come either from your congregation or from outside your church. Another option to having live speakers is to use the videos in the Bod4God Media Kit. These videos are designed to be a perfect complement to this book and are available at www.bod4god.org.

Step 3: Conduct Weekly Small Groups

Most participants will connect best with the program in their small group teams. Each team should choose a team name based on a fruit or vegetable as a rallying cry. During each team meeting, the participants should:

- Go over the information in this book chapter by chapter
- Specifically discuss the weekly Victory Guide assignments
- Share ideas on what works and what doesn't work for each person
- Cheer each other's successes
- Pray with each other

For more detailed information, see chapter 10.

Step 4: Conduct a Celebration

Although the weekly rally time is a kind of celebration, you want to have a big final rally celebratory event. Note that:

- During this last-week celebration, you will change the order of the meeting by having the small group time first and the rally time second. (The small groups will meet first to go over the material in week 12.)
- You will announce the overall weight loss for the group and the various teams during the celebration and recognize the individual biggest loser(s). Give each participant a certificate of participation (available at www.bod4god.org).
- You should decide if you would like to give out prizes.
- Any food for this event should be healthy.
- If you have individuals who have had unusual success, you may want to call in the media to do a story.
- You will want to rejoice over what God has helped you accomplish together. Make sure everyone leaves feeling like a winner.

START LIVING...START LOSING

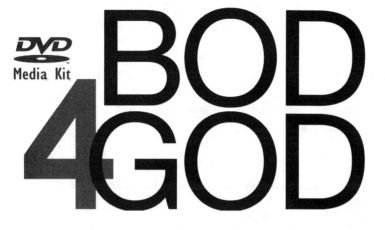

DVD Media Kit

BOD4GOD

FEATURES INCLUDE:

- COMPLEMENTS THE *BOD4GOD* BOOK.

- FOUR DVDS WITH TWELVE, 25-MINUTE VIDEO SESSIONS, PLUS GROUP STARTER TOOLS.

- EXPERT INTERVIEWS WITH DOCTORS, TRAINERS, NUTRITIONISTS, PASTORS AND PHIL AND AMY PARHAM (ON SEASON 6 OF NBC'S *THE BIGGEST LOSER.*

- TWELVE BOD4GOD THOUGHTS AND TESTIMONIES, ALSO 24 BOD4GOD FACTOIDS.

AVAILABLE AT
WWW.BOD4GOD.ORG

VIDEO PRODUCED BY INNOVATIVE FAITH RESOUCES

© LOSING TO LIVE. ALL RIGHTS RESERVED

ISBN: 978-0-578-09172-3

FOR MORE INFORMATION
VISIT WWW.BOD4GOD.ORG OR CONTACT

Losing to Live
P.O. Box 300
Merrifield, VA 22116
703-653-7100 • 866-596-6008

You may also contact Pastor Steve Reynolds about speaking to your church or organization

join first place 4 health today!

The First Place 4 Health Kit contains everything members need to live healthy, lose weight, make friends, and experience spiritual growth. With each resource, members will make positive changes in their thoughts and emotions, while transforming the way they fuel and recharge their bodies and relate to God.

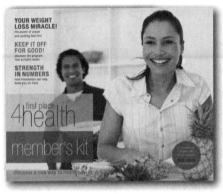

Member's Kit Contains:
- First Place 4 Health Hardcover Book
- Emotions & Eating DVD
- First Place 4 Health Member's Guide
- First Place 4 Health Prayer Journal
- Simple Ideas for Healthy Living
- First Place 4 Health Tote Bag
- Food on the Go Pocket Guide
- Why Should a Christian Be Physically Fit? DVD

978.08307.45890
$99.99 (a $145 Value!)

The First Place 4 Health Group Starter Kit includes everything you need to start and confidently lead your group into healthy living, weight loss, friendships, and spiritual growth. You will find lesson plans, training DVDs, a user-friendly food plan and other easy-to-use tools to help you lead members to a new way of thinking about health and Christ through a renewed mind, emotions, body and spirit.

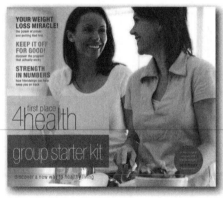

Group Starter Kit Contains:
- A Complete Member's Kit with Member Navigation Sheet
- First Place 4 Health Leader's Guide
- Seek God First Bible Study
- First Place 4 Health Orientation and Food Plan DVD
- How to Lead with Excellence DVD

978.08307.45906
$199.99 (a $256 value!)

www.firstplace4health.com